D1443156

Music

Music

THE NEW AGE ELIXIR

LISA SUMMER
WITH JOSEPH SUMMER

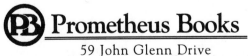 Prometheus Books

59 John Glenn Drive
Amherst, New York 14228-2197

.01001310
60113309

Published 1996 by Prometheus Books

00 99 98 97 96   5 4 3 2 1

Library of Congress Cataloging-in-Publication Data

Summer, Lisa.
    Music : the New Age elixir / Lisa Summer with Joseph Summer.
        p.   cm.
    Includes bibliographical references and index.
    ISBN 1–57392–104–1 (hardcover : alk. paper)
    1. Music therapy. 2. Music—Psychological aspects. 3. New Age music.
I. Summer, Joseph. II. Title.
ML3920.S88   1996
615.8′5154—dc20   96–2765
                                                                          CIP
                                                                          MN

Printed in the United States of America on acid-free paper.

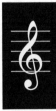

Contents

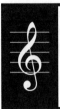

1. Preface: Right Alertness

dries Shah tells the story of Nasrudin, a Sufi master with a sense of humor.

> Nasrudin went to a mosque and sat down. His shirt was rather short and the man behind him pulled it lower, thinking it looked unseemly.
> Nasrudin immediately pulled on the shirt of the man in front of him.
> "What are you doing?" asked the man in front.
> "Don't ask me. Ask the man behind—he started it."[1]

The story illustrates the state of affairs of a group of practitioners who use sound and music for "healing." These practitioners, best described as New Age music healers, have created amongst themselves a philosophy which lacks clarity and logic. It has grown out of myths and legends, converted into "facts" in a parody of how science progresses. The foundations and axioms of New Age music healing are based upon wishes and fantasies which the practitioners in the field have agreed, perhaps unwittingly, to believe are facts. This agreement is protected by the apparent good intentions of the music healers. Because they wish to heal people, it appears mean-spirited to attack the foundations of their craft. The apparent goodness of the music healers' pursuit has muted criticism too long and allowed these practitioners to proliferate and promulgate their unsound medicine. There is protection in numbers; and the field grows as memories of its origins fade.

In 1988 I began an investigation of music healing theory and practice. As a music therapist I believed that the boundaries between music therapy and New Age music healing were becoming blurred, and that the two needed to be clearly differentiated. To my surprise I found music healers making extraordinary claims such as the ability to cure cancer with "subsonic frequencies," or to ameliorate AIDS with subliminal messages, or to end obesity with music that utilized "Pythagorean intonation."

> The secrets of sound and vibration have been harnessed by the medical profession who were very dubious at first but were impressed when results proved favourable. . . . Even back in 1963 Dr. Robert Cochran, leprosy consultant to the Ministry of Health and American Mission for Leprosy, sent a patient to St. George's hospital, Tooting, with legs so dreadfully ulcerated that it was thought amputation could only save the leg. Fortunately they called in . . . a Wimple Street Physiotherapist who agreed to treat her with a sound instrument . . . after 46 treatments she was cured. The instrument that he used was not, of course, the sophisticated instrument we use today but the basic principle was there and the results were actually shown. [2]

In the above quote Dr. Peter Guy Manners claims that a case of leprosy has been cured with a "cymatic instrument," a startling claim for a malady that, as of yet, is still deemed incurable by medical science. My investigation questions whether the therapeutic claims of music healers, such as Manners, are legitimate.

To arrive at the answers I constructed an eight fold path whose steps are: (1) "A Preface: Right Alertness," a step you have already begun in which my motivation for writing this book is offered; (2) "Praxis: Right

Speech," in which I explore the background and established practice of the New Age music healing movement in America within the larger context of New Age philosophy; (3) "Afflatus: Right Purpose," in which I discuss channeling and the role of the occult in the inspiration of musical creativity; (4) "Systems: Right Concentration," in which I criticize the reductionistic theories of New Age music healers; (5) "Acoustics: Right Understanding," in which I lay bare the fatal flaw of most New Age music healing philosophies, videlicet: a fundamental misunderstanding of the physical properties of sound; (6) "Vibrations: Right Effort," in which I evaluate the concept of sound as a healing agent and related mechanistic therapies (such as various entrainment theories); (7) "Research: Right Vocation," in which I show how the misunderstanding of the "scientific method" in research leads to the misapplication of findings, erroneous conclusions, and unsupported claims; and (8) "Testimonials: Right Conduct," in which I reveal how a lack of credible research or proven results is often obfuscated by unsupported testimony, anecdotal claims, and ad hominem arguments.

The vast majority of New Age music healing philosophy is fatally flawed by the oversimplification of complex psychological, physiological, acoustical, and musical phenomena.

Some music healers' powers are represented—generally by themselves—as encompassing vast ranges of human disease and failure. Dr. Jonathan Parker, president of Gateways Institute, has constructed an enterprise based on the selling of subliminal tapes. Over "inaudible" commands that he has authored he adds recordings of various kinds of music. According to Parker, "A special signal processor causes the subliminal message to precisely parallel the movement of the music or ocean, ensuring a strong, consistent subliminal message throughout the tape. [The] synchronized music [is] recorded in stereo to access whole brain learning by sending different messages to the left and right sides of the brain. Synchronized music enhances receptivity to subliminal messages."[3] Parker claims his tapes can reduce pain, cure substance abuse, and much more.

In his brochure "Discoveries through Inner Quests" Parker claims that a specific tape will "dissolve" a smoker's desire to smoke. "Subliminal messages," the brochure assures, "convince your subconscious mind that you are a non-smoker, and you become one."[4] Besides tapes for adults, Parker offers subliminal training tapes for children.

A competitor in the tape cure business is Howard Richman, who uses "no hypnotic, subliminal, or verbal suggestions" in his recorded piano music. His company, Sound Feelings, avoids making written claims of its own by sending out a photostatic and tinted copy of a newspaper article about Richman. The article reports that Richman "composes music to touch the fat or soothe the stress of overwrought adults . . . to heal the damaged psyche of small children." The article also makes the over-reaching claim that Richman is the progenitor of music therapy. "It was through Richman's interest in natural healing that the idea for therapeutic music was born."

The article reports that before Richman creates a piece, "he prepares himself by thoroughly researching the illness." He also reads of related work already done in the field of music healing, such as Steven Halpern's theory that each pitch of the C major scale corresponds to the seven levels of the body. Richman gently disputes Halpern, stating, "I would rather not say that music for fat people, for example, means I play a lot of D notes. . . . It's not as simple as that." He describes his *Feeling Stressed* tape as "intended to shatter your tension and . . . relieve general symptoms of stress, including those associated with coffee addiction, smoking, drinking, and drug abuse." Richman claims that the "sound chisels" of this twenty-two–minute tape will accomplish this feat. Richman's tapes include pieces titled "Cancer," "AIDS," and "Feeling Fat."[5]

Richman's claims are modest in comparison to some purveyors of subliminal message tapes. Potentials Unlimited distributes music/subliminal message tapes and other "therapeutic music" tapes under the headings "Astral Sounds" and "Music of the Spheres." Featured in its two-page promotional brochure is the "miracle" of Jennifer. The picture and story inform the reader that Jennifer was born three months premature weighing two pounds. She was not breathing and had to be "resuscitated." In addition, she was severely jaundiced, suffered from "debilitating seizures," and had fluid on her brain. Following the horrifying litany of Jennifer's profound diseases, the brochure proclaims that, "Jennifer's recovery isn't a miracle of spontaneous recovery, nor is it due to the intervention of medical technology." Her recovery is due to a series of four tapes developed by Jennifer's mother that Potentials Unlimited sells for $9.98 each. Barrie Konicor, the proprietor of Potentials Unlimited distributes the Jennifer tapes as well as many other subliminal tapes.[6]

Konicor's brochure advertises *Astral Sounds,* a tape which he claims "cannot be duplicated by the conventional tape duplicating equipment. Tapes duplicated on such equipment may sound similar to the original but will be ineffective. It requires our programmed computers to capture all of the sound waves needed to make *Astral Sounds* do what they are intended to do." This inability to duplicate the *Astral Sounds* tape is due, it is claimed, to the fact that the "sound frequencies . . . are so delicate, so exactingly accurate."

In language reminiscent of P. T. Barnum, Konicor notes that the tape recording is "truly unique. It is the only one of its kind in existence in the entire world." Konicor reports that hundreds of thousands of people use *Astral Sounds,* that hospitals use it "to tranquilize their patients instead of giving them sleeping medication. *Astral Sounds* can be used instead of a sleeping pill. Hospitals and Pain Centers use *Astral Sounds* to reduce or stop pain rather than use potentially dangerous pain-killing drugs. Colleges, Universities, and Boards of Education world-wide use *Astral Sounds* in their psychological programs. Heads of Government, Cabinet Members, and Supreme Court Justices use *Astral Sounds*."[7] Perhaps. But, neither Konicor nor Potentials Unlimited has made this evident through established medical journals.

Potentials Unlimited makes use of scientific-sounding language to bolster its claims. A "team of psychologists" is described as having programmed the tape, conjuring up images of professors in white lab coats surrounded by 1950s style IBM computers. "Sound waves and sound frequencies" are "arranged in a specific pattern," Konicor reports tautologically. "As soon as a person begins to listen to *Astral Sounds*, the sound waves immediately stimulate the small bones of the inner ear and vibrate the fluids of the inner ear's labyrinth." Apparently, the author of the Potentials Unlimited brochure felt that saying "you hear it," would not adequately describe the experience. This obscurantism may be necessary to disguise the basic unsoundness of Potentials Unlimited's claims, one of which is that people in an excited or euphoric state of mind actually produce sounds "inside their heads." This bizarre contention led Potentials Unlimited to "the ultimate scientific question . . . if feeling unusually healthy and happy mentally will result in these sound waves, will listening to an accurate duplication of these sound waves automatically make a person feel healthy and happy as well?" Obviously, an ultimate scientific question would interest scientists worldwide, and Konicor's *Astral Sounds,* it is claimed, was studied behind the "Iron Curtain" as well as by an unnamed "agency of the United States Government in Washington to discover why the listeners feel so perfectly healthy and happy every time they listen to *Astral Sounds."*

Astral Sounds, Konicor explains, is "an hour-long cassette fully copyrighted by The American Research Team." Though Konicor does not offer any explanation of just what comprises this "American Research Team," he does report their phenomenal results. "All test participants reported feeling better physically and emotionally after using the *Astral Sounds* tape cassette." Unanimous success is indeed a rare phenomenon in the testing done by medical research teams, but not impossible. Konicor's success rate may be due in part to the facility in which the taping was done, a "sound laboratory with a number of computers including a computer capable of creating any sound imaginable, known as a 'synthesizer.' " Konicor's research team, he claims, was able to faithfully duplicate each tone, pitch, and sound wave heard by the research subjects when they were in "an unusually happy, healthy and blissful state of mind," based on the subjects' descriptions of the sounds they were producing in their heads.

Astral Sounds, it is promised, will make worries, stress, anxiety, and pain disappear. Of special interest to the community of psychics is the report by Potentials Unlimited that the tape is used by many professional psychics "to make themselves even more psychic."[8]

Konicor clothes his unsupported claims in the garb of science, but they ring hollow, much like the pseudoscientific ramblings of B-movie mad scientists as they attempt to clarify badly scripted nonsense in verbose and inadvertently comic explanations. In the 1966 movie *The Vulture,* Eric, a nuclear physicist (played by Robert Hutton) explains to his brother-in-law (played by Broderick Crawford) how a giant werevulture has eavesdropped on sounds suspended "in the aether" for 250 years. If the following portion of the dialogue from *The Vulture* seems absurd, it is no more so than much of what passes for scientific explanations by sundry music healers studied in the following chapters.

E: Some unknown scientific brain has produced a monstrous creature—half bird, half man by means of nuclear transmutation. . . .

B: What is nuclear . . . uh, uh . . . transmutation?

E: The changing of atoms of one element to those of another by suitable nuclear reactions.

B: Would you put that in simple language?

E: A living person has been transferred through the aether and reassembled in the grave of Francis Real. Now, what was in that grave has, in a like manner, been transferred and reassembled in the place where the experiment was made.

B: Is this really possible?

E: Yes. Only something went wrong. Terribly wrong.

B: Oh? What's that?

E: Whoever made this experiment failed to take into account the vulture that was buried with Real and the threat to your family that was still in the grave.

B: Well, what are you trying to say now?

E: I'm not trying to say anything. Every sound ever uttered is still in the aether waiting to be recaptured. This unknown someone accidentally did it—recaptured the threat of a man buried alive.

B: And?

E: From the grave has come this creature with a threat to wipe out every member of your family from the youngest to the oldest, in that order: you; your brother, Edward; and Trudy.[9]

"As mysticism and science begin to blend more and more," begins Jonathan Goldman in his article on the "sonic healing arts" in the journal *Music Therapy.* This blending is exactly what is wrong in the field of music healing, an intrusion of unscientific gibberish in the garb of revelatory inner wisdom. An example of this blending is Goldman's citation of the story of "the One-hundredth Monkey," which, Goldman says, "explains that when a critical number of monkeys has learned to do a particular activity, this same activity is observed to be learned by another monkey on an island which is separated by many miles of ocean from the original group. The expansion of group consciousness is not limited by normal concepts of time and space."[10]

Often it is hard to know whether to take certain New Age gurus seriously. Are they teasing us? Testing our gullibility? Perhaps some are teaching a Zen lesson through purposeful misleading. Lyall Watson, a New Age sage, is famous for popularizing, indeed starting, the story of the "Hundredth Monkey." Here in his own words is the story:

One has to gather the rest of the story from personal anecdotes and bits of folklore among primate researchers, because most of them are still not quite sure what happened. And those who do suspect the truth are reluctant to publish it for fear of ridicule. So I am forced to improvise the details, but as near as I can tell, this is what seems to have happened. In the autumn of that year an unspecified number of monkeys on Koshima were washing sweet potatoes in the sea. . . . Let us say, for argument's sake, that the number was ninety-nine and that at eleven o'clock on a Tuesday morning, one further convert was added to the fold in the usual way. But the addition of the hundredth monkey apparently carried the number across some sort of threshold, pushing it through a kind of critical mass, because by that evening almost everyone was doing it. Not only that, but the habit seems to have jumped natural barriers and to have appeared spontaneously, like glycerine crystals in sealed laboratory jars, in colonies on other islands and on the mainland in a troop at Takasakiyama.[11]

However, Ron Amundson refuted Watson's story, debunking it as confabulated myth, and Watson replied to him (in part) by writing:

I accept Amundson's analysis of the origin and evolution of the Hundredth Monkey without reservation. It is a metaphor of my own making, based—as he rightly suggests—on very slim evidence and a great deal of hearsay. I have never pretended otherwise.

I take issue, however, with his conclusion that, therefore, the Hundredth Monkey Phenomenon cannot exist.

It might have come to be called the Hundredth Cockroach or Hairy Nosed Wombat Phenomenon if my travels had taken me in a different direction. As it happened, I was already interested in the nonlinear manner in which ideas and fashions travel through our culture, and the notion of quantum leaps in consciousness (a sort of punctuated equilibrium of the mind) was taking shape in my own mind when I arrived in Japan. It was off-the-record conversations with those familiar with the potato-washing work that led me to choose a monkey as the vehicle for my metaphor.[12]

Thus Watson admits that his "Hundredth Monkey Phenomenon" is nothing more than a fiction devised as a metaphor to explain a theory to support his way of thinking. It is a theory with no foundation in reality. There was never a ninety-ninth monkey or a one-hundredth monkey, washing potatoes, followed by a sudden explosion of potato washing amongst all of the monkeys of Koshima. Perversely, Watson's fiction has become, in many people's minds, established fact, and has been used as the basis for much New Age philosophy. This phenomenon of a confabulated theory actually contradicted by reality, yet used as the basis for further theorization (a house of cards, so to speak) is a feature typical not only of New Age philosophy but of the New Age music healers' theories of therapeutic music.

For the music healer, metaphor metamorphosizes into dogma, a phenomenon which might well be dubbed " 'The Hundredth Monkey Phenomenon' Phenomenon," in which, for instance, the music therapist's "iso principle" metaphor, in which the music therapist chooses music to match the psychological or physical state of their client, becomes the music healer's "factual" basis for belief that specific pitches can cure specific diseases. When the music therapist expresses an abstract idea, the New Age music theorist often misunderstands the abstraction as having taken place, much in the way that the New Age in general has latched on to the "Hundredth Monkey Phenomenon" as actual fact, rather than as the metaphor that Watson invented.

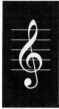

2. Praxis: Right Speech

A wanderer who ate rose-apples spoke thus to the venerable Sariputta:
"Reverend Sariputta, it is said: 'Nirvana, Nirvana.' Now what, your reverence, is Nirvana?"
"Whatever, your reverence, is the extinction of passion, of aversion, of confusion, this is called Nirvana."[1]

The Spiritual Canon

The New Age is an appellation used increasingly to describe a spiritual and cultural phenomenon that encompasses sundry beliefs and practices ranging from "ascended masters" conducting enlightenment exercises through correspondence courses to earnest and utile reexaminations of Western culture's prejudices and spiritual malaise. Its very name is misleading. How new is it? Corinne Heline (discussed later in this book) began publishing the *New Age Interpreter* in 1940. The *New Age Magazine* has been publishing monthly since before World War I. Perhaps the beginning of the New Age is 1875, when the infamous fraud and plagiarist Madame Helene Petrovna Blavatsky founded (with Colonel Henry Steel Olcott) the Theosophical Society.

Madame Blavatsky, a former piano teacher, made her fame channeling for a number of spirits. After successfully cultivating a group of seance clients with the noncorporeal guide, John King, and then with a posse of ancient Egyptians, Blavatsky struck psychic gold with an unprecedented (in the Occident) "partnership" with two ascended masters (or, as she often referred to them, Mahatmas), Koot Hoomi and Morya. These late Tibetan gurus would soon "dictate" from beyond the grave to Blavatsky two of the cornerstone books of New Age philosophy: *Isis Unveiled* and *The Secret Doctrine*, originally published in 1887 and 1888, respectively.[2] William E. Coleman, an early debunker of spiritualist buncombe, unveiled the ugly secret that both books were, for the most part, outright plagiarism, cribbed from several score other books; but whether Koot Hoomi and Morya or Madame Blavatsky were responsible for this theft, Coleman found no definitive proof.

The revelation of the plagiarism did not impede the growth of New Age movements (nor that of the Theosophical Society) and in the 1890s the World's Parliament of Religions imported numerous leaders and practitioners of oriental religions that proved so popular with the public that they took a permanent, if minimal, foothold on American soil. In 1894 Swami Vivekananda founded the Vedanta Society of America. Oriental spirituality had finally crossed the Pacific (in the flesh).

Whereas in Britain in the nineteenth century many members of the upper and middle classes had found an intriguing diversion in occult Egyptian spiritualism (note too, Madame Blavatsky's earlier and less successful spirit guides: the Brotherhood of Luxor's pharoanic visitors from the land of the Nile), American spiritualists favored the enlightened philosophies of China, Japan, and India. Chief among the oriental disciplines was Buddhism, the ancient offshoot of the even earlier Hinduism. Perhaps the multilimbed and metempsychotic deities of the Veda proved a trifle too fabulous for Americans. Buddhism, with its human progenitor, its inclination away from literal interpretation of the Vedas, and its superficial parallels to Christianity proved more attractive to the spiritualists and seekers of the early twentieth century. Now a peculiarly American notion of Hinduism/Buddhism is ineluctably associated with New Age philosophy and in many ways defines it.

New Age Buddhism reflects little of the philosophy of Guatama Buddha, but rather more of the philosophy of Madame Blavatsky. Proponents of the New Age are in revolt against what they see as inappropriate Western lifestyles and philosophy. Life should be a series of enlightening, joyful experiences, not a repressive and oppressive regimen of pain and penitence, proclaim many New Age prophets. In his teachings Buddha expresses his philosophy of pleasure:

> Let no man ever cling to what is pleasant, or to what is unpleasant. Not to see what is pleasant is pain, and it is pain to see what is unpleasant.
>
> Let, therefore, no man be attached to anything; loss of the beloved is evil. Those who are attached to nothing, and hate nothing, have no fetters.
>
> From pleasure comes grief, from pleasure comes fear; he who is free from pleasure knows neither grief nor fear. . . .
>
> From affection comes grief, from affection comes fear; he who is free from affection knows neither grief nor fear.[3]

Buddha's "Middle Way" eschews all pleasures, as is evident in this excerpt from the Fire Sermon:

> The ear is on fire; sounds are on fire; . . . the nose is on fire; . . . odors are on fire; . . . the tongue is on fire; tastes are on fire; . . . the body is on fire; . . . impressions received by the mind are on fire; and whatever sensation, pleasant, unpleasant, or indifferent, originates in dependence on impressions received by the mind, that also is on fire. . . . Perceiving this, O priests, the learned and noble disciple conceives an aversion for the eye, conceives an aversion for forms, conceives an aversion for eye-consciousness . . . conceives an aversion for the body, conceives an aversion for things tangible, . . . and whatever sensation, pleasant, unpleasant, or indifferent, originates in dependence on impressions received by the mind, for this also he conceives an aversion. And in conceiving this aversion, he becomes divested of passion, and by the

absence of passion he becomes free, and when he is free he becomes aware that he is free; and he knows that rebirth is exhausted, the he has lived the holy life, that he has done what it behooved him to do, and that he is no more for this world.[4]

The New Age practitioner who clings to pleasure is not a true Buddhist, but then the New Age has infused the concept of reincarnation with joy and pleasure, a kind of happy immortality. To Buddha, reincarnation was a bane, an educational experience to aid in accomplishing nonexistence. "Rebirth has been destroyed. The higher life has been fulfilled. What had to be done has been accomplished. After this present life there will be NO beyond!" In this portion of the Sammanaphala sultanta, Buddha yearns for a final freedom from existence. Life, he avers, is punishment.[5]

In pursuit of the musical elixir, it is common to find New Age healers relying on so-called Buddhist philosophy to justify their nostrums. One man's Buddhism is another's Budhism, as Madame Blavatsky explains to the "Enquirer" in her *Key to Theosophy*:

ENQ: What is the difference between Buddhism, the religion founded by the Prince of Kapilavastu, and *Budhism*, the "Wisdomism" which you say is synonymous with Theosophy?

THEO: Just the same difference as there is between the secret teachings of Christ, which are called "the mysteries of the Kingdom of Heaven," and the later ritualism and dogmatic theology of the Churches and Sects. *Buddha* means the "Enlightened" by *Bodha*, or understanding, Wisdom. This has passed root and branch into the *esoteric* teachings that Gautama imparted to his chosen *Arhats* only.

ENQ: But some Orientalists deny that Buddha ever taught any esoteric doctrine at all?

THEO: They may as well deny that Nature has any hidden secrets for the men of science. . . . His esoteric teachings were simply the

Gupta Vidya (secret knowledge) of the ancient Brahmins, the key to which their modern successors have, with few exceptions, completely lost.[6]

Whether or not Madame Blavatsky was a pretender to Orientalism, she was not ignorant, as she understood that Buddhism was not an Eastern version of Christianity. "One great distinction between Theosophy and exoteric [publicly revealed] Buddhism is that the latter . . . entirely denies a) the existence of any Deity, and b) any conscious post-mortem life, or even any self-conscious surviving individuality in man."[7] She acknowledged that this was the "purest" form of Buddhism, but added that Buddha had secret "esoteric" teachings that contradicted this.

The Musical Canon

Blavatsky's Theosophy, her esoteric teachings, profoundly affected two of her contemporaries, composers Alexander Scriabin and Cyril Scott, as well as Rudolf Steiner, a man whose theosophical offshoot, Anthroposophy, has had a marked influence on the New Age. Steiner's musical opinions provide a valuable insight into today's "Steiner influenced" music healers.

In the Bach family, the great-great-grandfather of Johann Sebastian was an individuality who lived on earth some fifteen or sixteen hundred years ago, when the human being was constituted quite differently. In Bach's grandfather another individuality was incarnated. The father is yet again a different individuality, and another incarnates itself in the son. These three individualities have absolutely nothing directly to do with the inheritance of musical talent. Musical talent is transmitted purely within physical heredity. The question of physical heredity is superficially resolved when we realize that man's musical gift depends on a special configuration of the ear. . . . This purely bodily basis for musical talent is handed down from generation to generation. We thus have a musical son, father, and grandfather, all of whom had musical

ears. Just as the physical form of the body—of the nose, for instance—
is handed down from one generation to another, so are the structural
proportions of the ear.[8]

Steiner's forays into music are but one small facet of his philosophy,
and his followers should have ignored his obviously untrue notion that
musical ability is connected to the structure, the shape, of the ear.
Beethoven composed when he was completely deaf. Were the shape of
his morbidly decaying ossicles still responsible for his genius? Steiner's
notion about musical ability we could ignore but for the strong influence
that his theories continue to hold today. This lecture, delivered on Decem-
ber 2, 1922, at Dornach seems to be the foundation of the work of Alfred
Tomatis, including Tomatis's peculiar and idiosyncratic view of the ear as
a "reflective organ."

Alfred Tomatis has built a theory of music healing upon the hypothesis that the ear itself is a battery that provides energy for the running of
the brain and body, and that certain specific sounds are necessary for
proper functioning. In Tomatis's view, for example, dyslexia is a disease
that can be ameliorated with the proper reception of specific frequencies
akin to the amelioration of certain "deficiency diseases" by the ingestion
of various vitamins.[9]

Where Steiner sees the physical construction of the ear as the home of
musical ability, Tomatis elevates the ear to the status of the alimentary system for the brain. This is akin to believing that specific colors as received
by the eyes literally feed the brain. I do not mean to imply that music or colors do not stimulate us. I object to the concept of these organs of reception
being erroneously classified as organs of digestion. What the ears hear and
the eyes see are transferred to the brain as nerve impulses, not calories.

Most music healers in search of a theosophically based precedent
have had to turn elsewhere for their musical theories. Alexander Scriabin
and Cyril Scott are the two competent composers most directly influenced by Madame Blavatsky. Both were acquainted with her personally.

Scriabin constructed a "history" of man and consciousness in the years 1907 and 1908. He called it "mysterium," and acknowledged his indebtedness to Blavatsky's theosophical theories for its formulation. Though he maintained a respect for Blavatsky even to the end of his life, Scriabin became disillusioned with Theosophy and eventually disposed of all other connections to it. His theosophical subscriptions remained unread, pages uncut. He considered Blavatsky's followers boors and culturally illiterate. It was particularly galling to him how little the theosophists understood or appreciated the fine arts, and music in particular. Scriabin complained of the English theosophists who attempted theosophical interpretation of his music and thereby to exploit him. "They do not understand, they do not understand, they do not love art."[10]

Boris De Schloezer's *Scriabin: Artist and Mystic* is a personal remembrance and intimate portrait of Scriabin. Given access to Scriabin's private writings De Schloezer includes notebook entries that reveal Scriabin in a nakedness that Scriabin may have resented, but display the narcissistic afflatus that drove him.

I want to enthrall the world by my creative work, by its wondrous beauty. I want to be the brightest imaginable light, the largest sun. I want to illumine the universe by my light. I want to engulf everything and absorb everything in my individuality. I want to give delight to the world. I want to take the world as one takes a woman. I need the world. I am what my senses feel. And I create the world by these senses. I create the infinite past, the growth of my consciousness, the desire to be myself. I create the infinite future, the repose in me, the sorrow and joy in me. I am God. I am nothing. I want to be all. I have generated my antithesis—time, space, and plurality. This antithesis is myself; for I am only what I engender. I want to be God. I want to return to myself. The world seeks God. I seek myself. The world is a yearning for God. I am a yearning for myself. I am the world. I am the search for God, for I am only what I seek. The history of human consciousness begins with my search and with my return.[11]

As accomplished an artist and brilliant a thinker as Scriabin was, he could engender no followers, no disciples, perhaps due to his charming, if foreboding, egotism. A man who sees himself at the center of the universe as Scriabin did often has little patience for the personal desires and needs of would-be apostles. "The ecstasy of Scriabin," writes De Schloezer, "averse as he was to struggle or tragedy, his absolute spirituality, his otherworldliness often seemed to be the marks of coldness and aloofness. The flaming world of Scriabin's mystique, too joyful and luminous for common comprehension, seemed to lack human warmth; ordinary people were dazzled by the blinding rays of Scriabin's sun and so could not enter his world."[12]

Notwithstanding the difficulty of approaching Scriabin on a personal or philosophical level, a substantial amount of his music is played and appreciated today and will be played and appreciated in the future, proving that at least some of his grandiosity and egotism was valid. Though Scriabin's music continues to be heard and he is generally acknowledged as the nonpareil mystic of classical music, he exerts surprisingly little influence on the world of New Age music. He is acknowledged by a few, but his desire for his music to be judged purely on its musical merits frightens away most music healers who believe that the effects of music on the listener have nothing to do with the composer's training, technique, or talent. Rather, music, even if vapid or unpalatable, needs only to contain the proper spiritual intent to succeed.

It fell upon composer/author Cyril Scott to forge a middle road between Steiner, the giant of Anthroposophy, whose musical knowledge was minimal, and Scriabin, the giant of mystical music whose interests laid in composition and not proselytization. Scott's music is nearly totally forgotten today, but his writings resonate through the pages of nearly all music healers' tomes. Through the years Scott's theosophical visions are reinterpreted by music healers, but ever so slightly; and his original contribution sometimes is adopted (without attribution) by the healer as his or her own. In 1989, a music healer who goes by the name Aeoliah wrote about how he saw the "future role" of "art and music ... in shaping the overall health of the Earth."

I ... see highly developed holographic concerts where the colors and lights will emanate from the musicians as they play the music. As the audience harmonizes with the event, the colors and lights from their auras will create resonant collective light images that will fill these huge pavilions and new concert halls with a beauty and harmony not yet experienced on the planet. Once the purity of the rainbow is rediscovered through the crystal chalice of the "collective consciousness of humanity," people will begin to surround themselves with only the purest pastel hues, or deeper more electric hues of more intense light frequencies. More iridescent mother-of-pearl hues and colors will be seen, rather than the drab greys and murky, muddy colors that have dulled the "collective aura" of humanity of the past. There will be more expanded light hues that will inspire, harmonize, and enhance any environment. Basically, a much more conscious use of color and sound will be incorporated in the mass consciousness of humanity, as these will help raise the energy level of each being into a higher octave of being and liberation.[13]

Preceding Aeoliah's vision by more than fifty years, Scott wrote, in the chapter "The Music of the Future" in his book *Music*:

Innovations will take place in connection with concerts. Already there have been complaints from the more fastidious music-lovers that concert-halls are too garishly lighted, and that what is seen detracts from what is heard. Such people, however, have usually been set down as cranks, and concert promoters have paid no heed to their idiosyncrasies. Nevertheless, the time will come when the demands of these so-called cranks will be fulfilled, and in an atmosphere of semidarkness colours of every variety will be projected on to a screen, expressive of and corresponding to the content of the music. Thus will that dream of Scriabin's be realised, the unity of colour and sound; and through its reali-

sation the audiences of the future will experience the healing and stimulating effects of that very potent conjunction.[14]

As Aeoliah claims his vision of the music of the future to be his own
original idea, something he saw in a vision, we cannot trace the true origin of his thought, whether it be from Scott back to Steiner, or directly
from Scott, or even possibly a variation of Scriabin's own ideas. Not all
New Age music healers claim spontaneous discovery (or rediscovery) of
theosophically derived visions. David Tame, a contemporary music healer/
theorist, is a scholarly writer who credits clearly the originators of the
ideas he discusses. Nevertheless, he does not attempt to demystify the
process and claims to draw ideas from the adept known as "El Morya,"
who, according to Tame "helped to form the Theosophical Society through
his chela, H. P. Blavatsky."[15] Tame considers the late Madame Blavatsky a
messenger of the Great White Brotherhood, and Tame believes that El
Morya has chosen new messengers for the continuing mission of the Great
White Brotherhood: Mark and Elizabeth Clare Prophet. Elizabeth Clare
Prophet is familiar to many people outside the New Age for her sophisticated weaponry armory at her cult's enclave in the Midwest.

El Morya, says Tame, will soon write the text to a grand theosophical
musical work with music written/channeled by Norman Thomas Miller.
Koot Hoomi, said Cyril Scott, channeled musical compositions through
Nelsa Chaplin, "a highly-trained clairvoyant of unusual sensitiveness.
who, since her earliest days had been in close telepathic contact with
Master Koot Hoomi"[16] Koot Hoomi and Morya were Madame Blavatsky's two principal channels. It seems that David Tame is assuming a
modern-day role as Scott, El Morya the role of Koot Hoomi, and Norman
Thomas Miller the role of Nelsa Chaplin. Tame's New Age is merely
duplicating New Age events which took place five decades ago, when
Nelsa Chaplin would sit at the piano, and

Master Koot Hoomi would actually play through her, when He desired to achieve some special—usually healing—effect on those under her care, for it should be mentioned that during a number of years she was associated with a species of guest-house which, in connection with her husband and a doctor, was run mostly for the treatment of strange and obstinate diseases, many of which had baffled more orthodox medical practitioners. A system of colour-healing had been evolved under the direction of the Masters, and very remarkable were some of the results achieved in regard to these diseases, which were usually found to be psychological in origin, and to involve the subtler bodies.[17]

Scott believed that Nelsa Chaplin not only channeled music for the theosophical spectre Koot Hoomi, but also that she was directly involved in healing through this music, sometimes with the aid of theosophically derived color therapy. In addition, Chaplin, as reported by Scott, experienced out-of-body experiences to aid in her spiritual healing (presaging the work of the contemporary music healer, Robert Monroe): "The Master Koot Hoomi and the Master Jesus frequently overshadowed [Chaplin] and used her as Their medium. She told me how . . . she had experienced the wonderful sensation of being lifted out of her body by Master Koot Hoomi, and how, as she stood by His side in her spiritual body, she saw Him controlling her physical [*sic*] in order to speak to her husband and the doctor."[18]

Like so many of today's music healers Scott saw his task as a divine mission guided by spirits from the past. Intriguingly, neither he nor his counterparts today ever question the wisdom of the "ancients." Accepting—for the sake of argument—the hypothesis of ascended masters speaking through channels, it is troubling that no music healer questions the credentials of the ascended ones or their motivations. Any voice from the past is obeyed unflinchingly simply because it is from the past. Though the New Age movement on the surface claims to look toward a better future, in reality it displays a severe conservatism in which the world never changes. Today's music healer wishes to practice therapy in the identical way that it has been practiced in the ever-receding past. What Koot Hoomi or El Morya defined as proper at the turn of the last century is considered the right path to follow now, and that only because they speak of the more distant past, spiraling backwards into mythical Atlantean civilizations preceding all written history. This strange nostalgic reverence creates a philosophy of healing frozen in time, so that what is said in 1990 is identical to what was said in 1890. And yet, the philosophy is often decorated with the word *evolution,* as in the ubiquitously repeated phrase, "spiritual evolution." Contrarily, the spiritual evolution is nowhere to be found. What is omnipresent is a worship of the status quo clothed in the garb of divine inspiration.

> My own association with Nelsa Chaplin extended over a period of seven years, and during that time on many occasions Master Koot Hoomi spoke to me through her, giving of His pearls of wisdom and instructing me as to how I could best serve the Great White Lodge, not only by my music—which He often inspired—but also by my pen. It was on one of these occasions that He told me the time had come when it was desirable that mankind should be enlightened regarding the esoteric effects of music and its influence upon well-nigh every phase of civilisation. "And it is for you, my son," He added, "to write a book on this subject, with the aid of the beloved pupil through whom I speak."[19]

In order to communicate with Cyril Scott, Koot Hoomi possessed the body of Nelsa Chaplin so that "the great philosopher and musician, Pythagoras the Sage" could write Scott's book.[20] (Pythagoras via Koot Hoomi via Nelsa Chaplin via Cyril Scott to the reader.) The backward spiral of channeled wisdom is not new to the 1990s. Wallowing in the past is a paramount feature of music-healing philosophy. But the vision of the past is clouded and fallacious. Outmoded, obsolete, and inaccurate science and technology are unearthed from their graves. These skeletons are dressed in pastel robes and presented as possessors of information necessary for our advancement.

The Scientific Canon

Imagine that you wish to explore new worlds, not of your inner psyche, not figurative new worlds; but real new worlds, Venus, Mars, or Jupiter. Assuming that you had the resources of NASA at your disposal, where would you go to plan your journey? With whose work would you construct a plan for your trip? Knowing that you need a useful solar system map, would you consult the writings of Galileo? No, he was brilliant, and advanced the knowledge of our solar system, but his map is flawed, his orbits circular, not ovoid. Naturally, you would consult the most esteemed astronomers of today, even should they be lesser minds than Galileo. Today's astronomers would make mistakes, too, but your journey's chances of success would be improved by using their less inspired but more accurate knowledge. Now, this is not to say that you would be safer to take along tapes of the Bee-Gees rather than Beethoven, but art is not science. This simple statement is a confounding confusion to New Age theorists, who are either incapable or unwilling to acknowledge the evident difference between art and science. Great art is not anachronistic. We can listen to Beethoven's Fifth Symphony and experience a gamut of aesthetic reactions today, but though we can admire the creativity and contributions of ancient scientists, we must, where their work is no longer adequate, dismiss their erroneous or misleading conclusions. Do we disprize Galileo for mistakenly assuming that the orbits of all celestial objects must be circular? No, but to claim they were, out of respect for Galileo, would appall Galileo as well as cripple your space program. In fact, the idea of worshipping the individual's contribution to knowledge such that it prevents improvements, emendations, or revisions is anithetical to the concept of science.

Echoing throughout the history of New Age music theory is the quest to validate Pythagoras's "music of the spheres" as pragmatic and utile theory, not the quaint poetic metaphor to which it has been relegated because of the advance of scientific knowledge. That Pythagoras believed the Earth to be the center of the universe and the planets in incorrect order (not to mention that in Pythagoras's construction the relative sizes of the celestial objects is all wrong) does not impinge itself upon the consciousnesses of those who view Pythagoras's theoretical musings on astronomical noise as relevant and true even today. Pythagoras's "music of the spheres" identifies the musical intervals of the "planets" according to his belief in their relative distances. The earth-to-moon interval is a whole tone. The moon to Mercury is a semitone. However, the planet Mercury is a far greater distance from our moon than the moon is from earth. From Mercury to Venus is another semitone according to Pythagoras (yet Venus is between the earth-moon dyad and Mercury.) From Venus to the sun is a minor third, but from Mars to the sun (remember that Mars is further from the sun than Venus, Mercury, and the earth) is but a whole tone. From Saturn to the fixed stars (but of course, they are not fixed) is again a minor third, though if we accept the minor third of the Venus-sun relation the true interval of Saturn to the nearest stars (Alpha Centauri and Proxima Centauri), the actual "interval" would be greater than a major millionth.

Kepler, too, calculated a music of the spheres.

> He built a schema (later disproven) of the solar system based on the concept of the five regular solids of geometry, a refinement of the Pythagorean musical spheres, but as Aristotle stated (and Kepler should have appreciated), "the statement that the motion of the celestial bodies causes a musical harmony . . . is quite ingenious but fails to tell the truth. . . . They [the Pythagoreans] assume that the velocities . . . represent the relationships of a musical harmony. . . . We are not conscious of it because we hear it from the moment we are born."[21]

Kepler and Pythagoras were scientific geniuses, but their contributions to knowledge must be looked upon in the light of further refinements and corrections.

When music healers resort to science it is often worse than when they do not. The science of sound (acoustics) is not their forte. Few music healers are competent in this field, yet few abstain from reckless hypothesizing in it. Many music-healing practitioners explain their healing art as based on sound acoustic principles, failing to heed the caveat issued by Rudolf Steiner in a lecture at Stuttgart in March 1923: "When it comes to acoustics, or tone physiology, there is nothing to be gained. Acoustics has no significance, except for physics. A tone physiology that would have significance for music itself does not exist."[22]

Many who otherwise appreciate Steiner's admonition nevertheless have chosen to latch on to the superficial aspects of the science of acoustics, seeing esoteric meaning behind the straightforward technologies of the acoustician. For them, an oscilloscope takes on magical properties. Like the primitive islanders of the cargo cult who worshipped planes as the manifestation of God, these music healers look on in awe at the patterns created by vibrations on the Chladni plate. In *Music*, Cyril Scott initiated an odd worship of the Chladni plates.

> It has been proved that sound can be both constructive and destructive: it can create forms, it can also destroy forms. From a chaotic sprinkling of sand on a glass plate, geometrical patterns may be formed with the aid of a violin-bow drawn across the edge of the plate, a fact which goes to prove the constructive effect of sound-vibrations. Conversely, the sound of the human voice may be employed to shatter a tumbler or wine-glass to atoms.[23]

Even in this relatively benign beginning to the worship of the Chladni plates, Scott misinterprets the phenomenon, fabricating a difference between vibrations caused by the human voice as opposed to those caused by a bow, whereas the difference is irrelevant to the examples given. Corinne Heline associated the patterns of the Chladni plate with an ill-defined process connecting heaven and earth. David Tame, Steven Halpern and Louis Savary, and Hazrat Inayat Khan are just some of the contemporary music healers who attribute esoteric meaning to the natural phenomenon demonstrated by the Chladni plates.

The Cultural Canon

A quality of secrecy, or esoteric meaning, is essential to the New Age music theorist. Devoid of secrecy, Western music, the music of Beethoven, Bach, and Brahms, is frequently held in disrepute, as being incompatible with humanistic, holistic healing. Objections to traditional Western music usually revolve around the notion that only the oriental musical traditions are truly healthy. Western music is too intellectual, not physical, not linked to the whole body as is the oriental musical tradition. Much of the music healer's music, they assert, is oriental in spirit. They claim to eschew the Western traditions in regard temperament, harmony, rhythm, and melody as traditional Western medical practice eschews acupuncture, herbal healing, and the like. The music healer believes that Western music lacks a proper, hence spiritual, oriental foundation necessary for healing purposes. Though traditional Western composers have always been interested in oriental influences, this influence has been, admittedly, minimal. Scarlatti captured Moorish influences in his piano music. Mozart and Weber wrote Turkish operas. Beethoven's Ninth Symphony includes percussion instruments first imported by the Turks into Europe. Wagner planned an opera based on Indian mythology. Bizet planned and completed an opera, *The Pearl Fishers,* based on an "Indian" story (though it is only marginally Indian). Puccini's *Turandot* is the story of a Chinese princess who believes she is the reincarnation of an abused predecessor, a subject also turned into an opera by Busoni. The twentieth century has seen hundreds of "oriental" Western pieces. Gustav Holst was especially interested in Indian folklore and religion, composing a Wagnerian style opera, *Sita*, based on the Ramayana and a smaller work *Savitri* derived from the Mahabharata.

Puccini's and Busoni's *Turandot*s make only token use of Chinese traditional music, using the pentatonic scale as a device to impart a Chinese flavor to otherwise clearly Western music. Holst does not attempt any ragas and Bizet restricts the Indian aspect to names and story. But as ethnomusicological studies became available and creditable, composers began to incorporate non-Western music practices into their music. Most restricted their borrowing to the music of their own countries. Bartok, Kodaly, Janacek, and Stravinsky incorporated Eastern European folk music into their own classical compositions; but they were composers, not solely ethnomusicologists. No controversy erupted when Busoni mistakenly used the English folk tune "Greensleeves" in *Turandot*. After all, Busoni was not claiming to be a composer of Chinese music, he was simply using a Chinese story as a vehicle for his music. Likewise Bartok's string quartets derive some material from Eastern European folk music, but they do not rely on any association with this music to succeed as string quartets. No serious classical composer has gone to great lengths to faithfully replicate non-Western musical traditions, nor made claims of any "superiority" in regard non-Western music. Their own unique imprimatur is always evident regardless of the influence of non-Western music. Puccini's *Turandot* is as evidently Puccini as is his *Madame Butterfly, Girl of the Golden West,* or *Tosca.* When Beethoven was commissioned to arrange over two hundred folk songs from the British Isles he did not simply transcribe the melodies, he infused them with Beethovenian qualities and a harmonic sophistication unknown in the originals. Again: Beethoven was a composer, not an ethnomusicologist. Bartok and Kodaly could perform their ethnomusicological duties and still create their own individualistic Western compositions. Nor did they disdain Western tradition.

The Psychological Canon

The New Age, protests notwithstanding, is infatuated with behavioral and simplistic solutions. New Age periodicals are replete with articles and advertisements wherein solutions to psychological and physical problems are addressed behaviorally, camouflaged in a vocabulary of holism. Companies advertise tapes that promise to reduce your stress, make you thin, accelerate your learning, heal your maladies, and get you rich, all without effort or conscious understanding. New Age music healer Steven Halpern asserts that the average person should not know about the processes involved in his healing. At the 1988 Music and Health Conference in Kentucky, Halpern stated, "We don't have to tell people exactly what we're doing. We don't have to tell them that we are going to heal them by showing them certain colors or playing them certain sounds. . . . Depending upon the semantic materialism that Don [Campbell] was mentioning about last night, we may just couch our terms in less confrontational aspects."[24]

To Halpern and not a few of his brethren, understanding the process of healing is too "confrontational." Some music healers deplore confrontation and personal contact so much, they refrain from any contact other than the mailing of cures and the acceptance, again through the mail, of checks. In an age where the paucity of doctors who will make house calls is bemoaned, it is odd that some people are satisfied to be attended by healers whose faces they never see, whose hands they never touch; healers who never hear their complaints or explanations, but who merely send their patients cassettes.

"The tapes are outstanding! I am working with them daily with remarkable benefits. I love the way he [Jonathan Parker] serves everything on a silver platter," enthuses B. P. of Florida about Parker's subliminal tapes series.[25] Parker's Gateways Institute hawks several dozen tapes with titles such as *Freedom from the Use of Alcohol, Freedom from the Use of Drugs, Stop Smoking, Sleep Like a Baby, Look Young! Feel Young!, Weight*

Loss, Attracting Wealth and Prosperity, Successful Sales, Drug Prevention for Young People, Bring Laughter into Your Life, and even *Creativity.* The tapes are offered with a choice of music including "Easy Listening," "Contemporary Rhythm," "Romantic Moods," and "The Classics," as well as sound tapes of "Gentle Winds" and "Tropical Ocean."[26]

In Gateways Institute's brochure "Discoveries through Inner Quests" (which features a cover illustration of several planets, including Jupiter—à la Stanley Kubrick's film *2001*—approaching syzygy above a verdant mountain), the institute's director addresses the seeker of discoveries as a dear friend, and invites him to become transformed and illuminated, to attain a "higher consciousness," to uncover ancient secrets and release psychic powers. Gateways Institute promises these accomplishments can be obtained simply by listening to subliminal tapes.

To change behavior without considering the meaning of the change is Gateways Institute's modus operandi. Its ability to do this is another issue. The morality and propriety of changing behavior without attending to the holistic causes of the undesired behavior is yet another issue.

Potentials Unlimited is another subliminal tape company, with promises identical to Gateways Institute (though Potentials Unlimited is the only subliminal tape company I've discovered that claims to be able to improve your racquetball game). With a complement of some two hundred tapes, Potentials Unlimited claims that some of their tapes have remarkable healing properties, including the ability to cure "Cerebral Palsy [*sic*].[27]

Dr. Tim Lowenstein, the director of the Conscious Living Foundation, claims that his subliminal tape series of about one hundred tapes can cure stress and more. In addition to shopping his tapes he makes personal appearances where participants can "witness an amazing self-healing demonstration by Dr. Tim Lowenstein as he takes an ordinary safety pin and drives it deep into his arm. THERE IS NO PAIN! THERE IS NO BLEEDING!"[28] This common staple of the magician's bag of tricks is regularly performed on stages worldwide by performers who do not claim it to be healing. The magician Teller of the Penn and Teller duo performs this stunt with one major difference: he uses blood capsules to simulate the appearance of bleeding, as it makes for a greater theatrical effect.

Needle stunt aside, Lowenstein shares the same behavioral approach to a wide variety of illnesses and conditions as those of Gateways Institute and Potentials Unlimited. Many New Age music healers emulate this shallow behavioral approach, but eschew the subliminal message component, claiming that the music itself will work behavioral miracles. Howard Richman created the corporation Sound Feelings to distribute his tapes, which he claims ameliorate conditions of obesity, AIDS, and cancer; however, Richman is careful to include a medical disclaimer with his dubious offerings. Though Richman has been selling his tapes for many years, in 1980 he began to associate his curative music with entrainment.

> The music that I compose is with [*sic*] the express intention of bringing about the three qualities of entrainment: (1) to resonate or lock-in with the listener's present feelings; (2) to assist in the transformation of negativity into positivity; and (3) to arrive at a state of liveliness or serenity.
>
> The musical element most associated with entrainment is rhythm. However, if one really considers it, every component of music may be defined as a rhythm: pitch frequency, dynamic variation, harmony, phrasing, articulation. Each have a periodicity or rhythm. So it is really *all* elements of music that can entrain the listener.[29]

Though Richman claims that he infuses his music with "entrainment" qualities, he neglects to explain how he can "resonate or lock-in with the listener's present feelings" through the mailing of his tapes, as he is neither present nor aware of the individual listener's feelings. Does he mean to imply that his music will affect all people or, for example, all obese people, identically? This presupposes that all obese people suffer from the same etiology of obesity, and that upon receiving his tape, they will all listen to it in the same state of mind. Elsewhere in his literature Richman remarks that "you can't make one piece of music for everybody." But then, he also contradicts his assertion that his method of composition is scientific and purposeful when he writes that he composes, in actuality, not "with an analytical mind, I do it from a very deep and intuitive place."[30]

The most successful New Age subliminal tape salesman is probably Dick Sutphen, whose *Master of Life* periodical is forty pages of advertisements for sundry Sutphen merchandise, and five to ten pages of articles by or about Sutphen and his family. Sutphen's catalogue offers subliminal video and audio tapes with the same claims as those previously mentioned, only at generally higher prices. Titles include *Ultra-Monetary Success, Stop Biting Fingernails,* and *Higher-Self Finger Talk.* Sutphen shares a disregard for victims of tragedy with New Age guru Shirley MacLaine. In issue 38 of *Master of Life* Sutphen explained that victims of AIDS "predestined" their own illness "as a karmic balance."[31] In *Dancing in the Light* MacLaine wrote, "We are not victims of the world we see. We are victims of the way we see the world. In truth, there are no victims. There is only self-perception and self-realization."[32] If Sutphen's subliminal tapes are the most successful of their genre in New Age behavioral therapies, to what does he owe this unparalleled good fortune? Perhaps it is Sutphen's remarkable ability to advertise and promote himself as few others do or can. In a response to an inquiry regarding his possible background in advertising, Sutphen huffily responds,

Number one: I am whoever you think I am. How could I be anything else? Number two: Advertising is the most moral of all professions since it never pretends to be anything other than what it is. I've met a lot of New Age people and practitioners who claim spiritual enlightenment, but who can't honestly make that claim.

Note: Your handwriting shows great anger and frustration. Instead of worrying about my spirituality, you might be better served to look within for what you think you see in me that you recognize in yourself. We are all mirrors for each other.[33]

Masters Sutphen et al. restrict their subliminal message tapes to humans, but Noah's Ark Productions makes subliminal training recordings for animals. Their subliminal script, "How Much Is That Doggie in the Window?" which is meant to be played for your dog, admonishes, in first-person singular:

Send the sunshine of wisdom to guide me in my happy time of achievement. Help me to fashion my mental control so that I will not be distracted from my task or master. My sole thought is to my master's guidance. . . .
Lie down. Stay. I may feel scared, but I am calm. I will lie down and stay when asked because I may not see a car and my master and friend will protect me by telling me to lie down and stay. . . .
Eating. I will only eat what my master gives to me.
Chewing. I will chew only what my master gives me because I may choke and not be able to do my service. . . .
Teach me to consider no other duty more important than my master's commands since my work of any kind is possible only because thou has given me the power of performance.[34]

The inclusion of animals in New Age practices is not surprising. Animals and objects have become important fetishes in New Age culture. Fetishism is often considered the worship of objects, but is best defined as

the friendly intercourse between man and the spirits that are supposed to inhabit these objects. . . . Fetishism falls right in line with modern superstitious beliefs and behaviorism. . . . A fetish is . . . a material object believed to be the dwelling of a spirit, or to be the representation of a spirit, which may be induced or compelled to help the possessor. Primitive animism, however, evolved into fetishism, and fetishism is the first step toward idol-worship. When we idolize a human being in an extreme sense, as such fanaticism expresses, that hero or heroine becomes part of modern fetish-worship."[35]

Whereas the Buddhist monk disdains the physical and its outer trappings, adorning himself in the simplest accoutrements, the New Age has its special costumes and fashion accessories. Chief among these is the crystal. Why the crystal has become the central fetish of the New Age has little to do with its actual properties, of which many New Age gurus are ignorant. Laeh Maggie Garfield, a New Age music healer, notes, "Quartz crystals are mainly composed of silicon dioxide—the same chemical that human beings are made of. This is a match-up in terms of energetic similarity, which might account for why every type of quartz is employed worldwide in healing people."[36]

Either Garfield did not pay attention in biology class or she is not talking about human types of people. Obviously, human beings are not made of silicon dioxide. Garfield is attempting to rationalize a common New Age ritual wherein a person "energizes" a crystal, usually for the purpose of healing. Quartz crystals resonate at millions of cycles per second. Human brain wave patterns do not exceed 1,000 cycles per second. In addition, human brains do not produce sufficient electrical power to cause a crystal to vibrate. To "energize" a tiny crystal would take a minimum of one thousand people. The amount of wire necessary for such an operation depends upon how many people you could crowd around the accumulator. That crystals have long held a cherished place in human society is true, but so has the dog and few New Age gurus are championing dogs as reservoirs of spiritual power.

Dogs, however, do get lost when you don't keep them on a leash or train them properly, which property they do not share with crystals, though Laeh Garfield would disagree. "Crystals disappear," writes Garfield. "Crystals will leave you if they do not belong with you. The Tule Indians say that if you lose a crystal, do not go hunting for it. If it's yours, it'll come back to you. If not, it belongs to the finder and you mustn't ask for its return. They will literally jump out of your hand if they aren't meant for the healing you are about to do. And they'll fall from your pocket or hand at other times if they're meant for another person."[37]

Unlike lost dogs, however, Garfield can "rematerialize crystals because I wanted them back so badly. And you can probably do the same with a bit of practice."[38] This talent could prove very valuable to larcenous jewelers. They could rematerialize diamonds recently sold (but only if they wanted them badly enough.)

As Claudia De Lys explained, fetishism can extend to human beings, and it does so in the New Age music field wherein music healers deify composers from Wagner to themselves, imbuing the human with spirits that inhabit these composers.

Cyril Scott asserts that Wagner was inhabited by "Devas"; Cesar Franck was "closely in touch with the Deva-evolution."[39] Scriabin, however, was "not a trained Initiate working under the supervision of a Master; and hence in contacting the Devas of the higher planes, he subjected his delicate physical vehicle to such a strain that he laid himself open to the attacks of the Dark Forces."[40] Scriabin's failure to keep the Dark Forces at bay caused his premature death, according to Scott. Presumably, Scriabin's distaste for Blavatsky's followers had no bearing on Scott's opinion of Scriabin.

Corinne Heline wrote that, "Richard Wagner was an inspired musical Initiate who knew how to attune himself to the mighty powers directed earthward."[41] She also deified Bach, describing him as a high priest of music and a channel from the "highest heaven (the third heaven of Paul). . . . To one seeking to obey Paul's injunction concerning the Christing of the mind, the music of Bach is all-important."[42] These attitudes are no different than contemporary forms of hero-worship that focus on singers, athletes, and movie stars. Hero-worship allows the fan to experience temporary feelings of security and ecstasy considered abnormal outside the boundaries of the fetish. Behavior tolerated at a Star Trek convention or Madonna concert would be considered unacceptable in daily conduct. Today, one of the most extreme forms of this fetishism is Elvis-worship, which subject could (and does) fill another book. How different is Heline and Scott's worship of Wagner from Elvis-worship? The Elvis fanatic sees in Elvis superhuman, deific qualities. Scott and Heline see the same qualities in Wagner.

Steven Halpern, disdaining the hero-worship of other composers, unapologetically attributes Deva-inspired qualities to himself. In an interview with himself that he records in *Tuning the Human Instrument*, Halpern asks himself, "Where on Earth does the [your] music come from?" He answers,

> Isadora Duncan had an answer for that that went something like, "Not from Earth, my dear, but from Heaven." That's how it feels for me. That's actually an interesting hypothesis, especially in light of recent research on interacting energy fields and resonance phenomena based on vibrational harmonics. Also, based upon a literary tradition which traces its heredity back to the legendary Muses, it wouldn't be the first time that an artist or poet or musician acknowledged some higher, divine Inspiration and cooperation.[43]

The New Age music healer/composer, as epitomized by Steven Halpern, faces a polyemma that composers like Beethoven eluded. Beethoven had a single difficulty, which was singularly abstract: to write good music. He did not need to question his inspiration, his motivation, or the possibly ameliorative effects of his craft. The New Age music healer/composer, however, faces the multiple task of writing music that is universally palatable and universally palliative, as well as defending his craft on the grounds of a proper spiritual, scientific, and psychological (or parapsychological) foundation. What we perceive as pomposity in Halpern is, in fact, a necessity and the principal justification for the pursuit of his goal: music that heals. Prior to putting pen to paper, or hand to electronic keyboard, the New Age music healer imposes upon himself the precondition that what he writes is not merely a pleasant or rewarding piece of music, but rather a prescription for health.

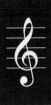

3. Afflatus: Right Purpose

Wouldst thou be good, then first believe that thou art evil.

The beginning of philosophy, at least with those who lay hold of it as they ought and enter by the door, is the consciousness of their own feebleness and incapacity in respect of necessary things.

For we come into the world having by nature no idea of a right-angled triangle, or a quarter tone, or a semi-tone, but by a certain tradition of art we learn each of these things. And thus those who know them not, do not suppose that they know them.[1]

Unearthly Inspiration

Inspiration is often the rationale given to explain the creative process of the great composer, a deus ex machina of afflatus where great music floats down from the welkin to drip through the pen of the medium of the message. In actuality, Mozart wrote great music while talking with friends or playing skittles. Beethoven's inspiring angels must have been very flighty indeed as he sketched the opening of his Fifth Symphony a hundred different ways before finding the properly inspired immortal motto. His nonpareil last movement to the *Choral* Symphony began life as the far less lofty *Choral* Fantasy, opus 80, in which the choral hymn makes a premature and unfinished appearance. Every composer has a method for the construction of his music, some more prosaic than others, but the reality of composition is that the composer who needs wait for inspiration is an exception to the rule, popular myths notwithstanding.

Composers themselves encourage the myth of divine inspiration. The twentieth-century composer Pfitzner in his opera *Palestrina* depicts the eponymous composer receiving the music to his most famous mass in dictation from angels. Pfitzner's reconstruction of Palestrina's *Mass* is an intellectual exercise, his use of Palestrina's music precise and contrived. Pfitzner creates the illusion of spontaneous generation through his own careful pedantic preparation. "Ars est celare artem" is the Latin phrase that so accurately illuminates Pfitzner and all great composers' works: the art consists in concealing the art. Though Beethoven may have struggled to strike the right chord for the Fifth, the listener must not know this. The process of the composition must not be revealed. The listener is allowed to hear only the final reification of the composer's labors.

Many New Age healer/composers deny that their music is constructed in the artificial way that Beethoven constructed his. As Athena sprang from Zeus's head so flow the pieces that they claim as theirs; or in self-proclaimed humility they admit that they are but the servants of higher powers, of angels, vedas, higher masters, and ethereal beings who must express themselves through mortal vessels.

These New Age music healers who transcribe the ideas of superior or unearthly agents follow in the path of Rosemary Brown, the matriarch of musical channelers, whose work, if valid, would make irrelevant another Latin motto of note: "Ars longa, vita brevis," "Art is long, life is short."

Rosemary Brown, a self-described "ordinary housewife" from a poor suburb in London, began receiving spiritual visitations from Liszt at the age of seven (in the 1930s), to which she claims she attached no special importance. However, in 1961, Liszt offered the newly widowed and impoverished Brown "real practical help."

"Easter came around," writes Brown in her autobiographical *Unfinished Symphonies*, "and . . . I was at my wit's end to think how to manage

. . . Liszt then said most unexpectedly: 'I think that perhaps you should try the football pools this week.' " To Brown's "astonishment" she won ten pounds. The following Christmas Liszt "again suggested, with a little twinkle, that I might just try the pools again. I took his advice, and this time the dividend was 51 odd."[2] Liszt was not done twinkling for Rosemary Brown. In 1964, Liszt began dictating music to her, and then began serving as leader of a group of famous composers who visited her at her home and dictated to her their "new" compositions. The group comprised the twelve composers: Liszt, Chopin, Schubert, Beethoven, Bach, Brahms, Schumann, Debussy, Grieg, Berlioz, Rachmaninov, and Monteverdi.

Several of Brown's channeled transcriptions were recorded in 1970, revealing that the deceased composers' skills had deteriorated from their heights of genius. British composer Richard Rodney Bennet defended the mediocrity of the works in his commentary, "Even if some of the pieces are bad, that doesn't mean anything. I produce lots of lousy pieces."[3] But one is compelled to question why Liszt would wish to resurrect himself with samples of barely credible juvenilia after all those years (but then, how does time progress after death?) in the afterlife. Interestingly, all the composers' pieces show remarkable signs of deterioration. Those that retain any similarity to the supposed composer's style seem pale, music-student improvisations, including the harmonically jejune showpiece of Brown's collection, Liszt's *Valse Brilliante* (two pages of which Brown unwisely includes in the book *Unfinished Symphonies*). But then this may only be evidence of the common activity all these composers have shared since their deaths, namely: decomposing.

A fund was established for Brown in 1968 to free her from work so that she could devote herself full time to transcription, and expectations arose of symphonic works. The expectations exceeded the faltering capabilities of her spirit composers. With Brown's channels no longer communicating their musical inventions to her, her fans and followers left her. The fund stopped funding her, and even Liszt became listless and ceased dictating to her. But do not mourn Brown, she may return yet. During her heyday, Sir George Trevelyan, one of the two trustees of Brown's fund, wrote, "In the present critical human situation it might well be that the higher worlds intended to use music as a redemptive and healing force."[4] Could not Brown's mission be resurrected? True, musicians, audiences, and critics ridiculed Brown's opera, but in a unique and brilliant defense of her verity and righteousness, she enlisted the aid of one of Britain's most eminent music critics, Sir Donald Tovey, who wrote in 1970,

> As you listen to this record [*A Musical Séance*], you may wonder whether the music you hear is the product of Rosemary Brown's abilities, or whether it has indeed emanated from departed composers who are still creating music in another world. This music has already called forth some admiration and some denigration, but I am happy to note that the former considerably outweighs the latter. I also note that those who denigrate the music usually do so, not as a result of certain exacting standards, but as the outcome of a measure of scepticism.[5]

Sir Tovey's defense of Brown, which appears on her album and in her book, is more remarkable for the fact that he made these comments thirty years after his death. Tovey's comments were made the night of January 1, 1970, to Brown while she was having trouble falling to sleep. According to Brown, Tovey was planning to dictate through her a post-mortem book entitled *Immortality*.

Debussy once remarked to Brown that since his death he'd taken up painting. Debussy could study with Schoenberg, who painted while alive. Otherwise he may have to wait for the earthly desinence of Aeoliah, a New Age composer/painter whose philosophy is revealed in the spring 1989 issue of *Halo*, a Canadian New Age magazine. In that issue several of Aeoliah's symmetrical portraits of white, blond men and women with big cat eyes are reproduced, in color. "Aeoliah" was not Aeoliah's given name.

As the name Aeoliah started to manifest within me, I became aware of my training in ancient Greece and Atlantis, where light, color and sound were a powerful dynamic expression of perfect Divine Harmony and Union with the cosmos. This music and these crystalline colors and light were projected directly in places we now call healing temples. One would stay in one of these rooms for perhaps half an hour and become totally healed, reintegrated, rejuvenated and revitalized. The sounds, light and color vibrations did not emanate from a machine or a mechanical recording device, but from beings of higher intelligence who projected this harmonious energy from the various chakras.[6]

I am unsure where, whether Greece or Atlantis, the Indian chakra healing took place; but Aeoliah's confusion regarding history and fiction pales beside his crystalline fetishism. "Scientists have recently discovered in our cerebro-spinal fluid a substance known as piezo-electric crystals which transmit and generate a tremendous amount of energy and information through electrically-charged impulses to the brain and various other centers in the body."[7]

Sometimes, Aeoliah takes personal credit for his music.

Every piece of music or every album I have recorded is a direct manifestation of a certain state in my evolution. Each album expresses a major turning point in my evolving awareness of self and how I view the world around me. This includes relationships with other people, marriage, divorce, children, the pain of separation, my sexual identity, the bliss of transcendental union with my Higher Self, my major emotional and psychological breakthroughs and, most recently, the major restructurization [sic] of limiting perception patterns and habits and my relationship to the world. All these events are catalysts that open up a new area in my being and psyche that allows the new music to come through. During this process of creation, a tremendous alignment of cosmic energy takes place that transforms my thinking process and my perceptions. The music that is being created is simultaneously empowered with these new energies, which then become a living universal reality for others as they experience the music. That is the main nature of the music I create—to allow each person the choice to hear that music as an expression of his or her own life essence as they experience the various stages of unfoldment, self-allowance, surrender and empowerment.[8]

Yet, paradoxically, Aeoliah also claims to be nothing more than a channel for "an energy and Being named Aeoliah," who was part of a "group of evolved beings," who "project their harmonious healing vibrations directly to any person, life form, or place, depending on the need of the moment."[9] Unlike many other New Age channels it appears that "Aeoliah" has become the channel for the eponymous Aeoliah, not just a performer or entertainer.

First of all, I would like to clarify the difference between being a performer and being an instrument for the healing process. So many of our musical events have been categorized as entertainment with performers entertaining the audience. This, to me, is an old concept and a very limited role for a musician to play. This role also carries with it a lot of stress to satisfy the audience, or to give the audience what they like to hear, or what makes them laugh. Again, this sets up a very linear goal-oriented process in which the precious beauty of a silent moment of one's own reality becomes lost or disturbed. You can also observe how this linear pattern creates a deliberate expectation on the part of the audience to be fulfilled from something outside of themselves. This is the main difference between the old concept of the entertainment-performer role and what takes place during my concerts. There is no entertainer, no performer, only a channel that is guiding the audience into the inner chambers of their own inner sanctums.[10]

"Aeoliah," the channel for Aeoliah, becomes the channel for the audience. Speaking of his music he writes, "The highest form of music is pure sound therapy."[11] Furthermore, "The music of 'Crystal Illumination' is transmitted through each [chakra] center, directly activating a balanced use of piezo-electric crystal substance which is released into each energy center. That is the 'Crystal Illumination' that takes place on a biochemical and wholistic level."[12]

Aeoliah claims that his music has the potential to heal our whole planet, as well as the cosmos. He believes that the media promotes an inharmonious music which "keeps the listener imprisoned in an astral world of fear and aggression."[13] I am unsure of what he means here by "astral world" as Aeoliah elsewhere approves of music that moves the listener to an "astral world," unless perhaps he means that there are bad astral worlds as well as good ones.

Aeoliah's writing is replete with misinformation culled from other New Age sources. Mixing tabloid facts with his own divinely inspired philosophy, Atlantean folklore becomes entangled in references to the Hindu religion, technological uses of crystals are transplanted without care into explanations of human physiology, and, like Rosemary Brown's defenders, those who protest inaccuracy and confusion are labeled pejoratively as skeptics. Skeptics' motives are questioned, whereas music healers' motives are not.

At issue is responsibility. Is a flagrant disregard for cultural and scientific facts irrelevant to New Age philosophy or is it a fundamental flaw in reasoning, and an admission of a logical bankruptcy? Too often the New Age music healers seem to be aware of the questionable merits of the scientific underpinning of their musical theories, only to abruptly evade the issue by paradoxically claiming supernatural approval for their musical elixirs. Music healers fail to see that their appeals to science are diametrically opposed to their appeal to faith.

When Aeoliah speaks of his music energizing piezo-electric crystals in our brains he lays bare the bankruptcy of his understanding of neurophysiology. Concurrently he complains that the scientific model is a hindrance to spiritual enlightenment. Why then does Aeoliah call upon scientific justification (in the form of his piezo-electric crystal chatter) to justify the efficacy of his music's ability to heal? As odd as it seems, Aeoliah himself is more trapped in the Western tradition than the musicians he attacks as spiritually unenlightened. Whether it is Beethoven or the latest pop composer, the artist generally creates his music without regard for scientific justification for his work. Aeoliah seems to need a rationalistic justification for his artistic endeavors. For Aeoliah this comes in the form of pseudoscientific theorizing combined with the claim of divine guidance. Aeoliah cannot be questioned. He says that the responsibility for his music lies not with him, but with piezo-electric phenomena or from ascended masters from the Atlantean past.

The call of Atlantis to the New Age music healer is powerful, and several other music healers claim the fabled continent as the source of their compositional abilities. Aeoliah and his ilk praise the scientific and technological accomplishments of Atlantis while berating today's scientists for attempting to create a real technological utopia. Peter Guy Manners illustrates his mystical reverence for a technology he does not understand when he imputes mystical significance to a technological device (the oscilloscope) in the same manner as a member of a primitive tribe, upon his exposure to an advanced technological artifact such as the radio, might infer that a god lives within the black box.

> If one takes an oscilloscope dialed to a polar coordinate system, and plays combinations of harmonics of F, the lissajous figures which result are beautifully structured linear diagrams of the sounds heard. One can do this by attaching an amplified speaker and microphones, or tape recorder to the oscilloscope in the proper manner. Inharmonious sounds to F in general would be G, E, B. The reason for this is that both E and G are so close to one another stepwise in the scale. . . . If you put an array of nonharmonically equivalent sounds on a matrix you would see how far apart these sounds would be from the origin of the diagram. Now the matrix I am speaking of goes back to ancient times, certainly to Pythagoras, but most probably to ancient Egypt and before that Atlantis and Lemuria. It is believed by many that these ancient peoples understood

better than we do today the components of light and sound, and made use of this to heal and in general benefit humankind of those ages.[14]

Manners's confusing mixture of science (the oscilloscope) with science-fiction (Atlantis) is typical in New Age music healing literature. A science-fiction author improves the believability of his fiction by accurately depicting scientific reality and then extrapolating a plausible extension into the future, but the reverse is not true. When discussing science, references to fantasy and illusion serve only to weaken and cast doubt upon a hypothesis. One cannot meaningfully support the plausibility of antigravity machines by claiming that such have been proven valuable instruments of travel in the movie *Star Wars*. This abuse of a priori assumptions is typical of many New Age music theories, which are often merely bald assertions of fantasy adorned with scientific-sounding gobbledygook. A recurrent theme is the music healer's reliance upon scientific information channeled from the fictional Atlantis. Numerous theories are supported by the work of Atlantean technological geniuses whose work is believed to be submerged beneath the waters of the Bermuda Triangle. Shakespeare's refutation of this muddled thinking is pithily given in act 3, scene 1, of Shakespeare's *Henry IV, Part 1*:

Glendower: I can call spirits from the vasty deep.
Hotspur: Why, so can I, or so can any man;
              but will they come when you do call for them?
Glendower: Why, I can teach you, cousin, to command
              the devil.
Hotspur: And I can teach thee, cuz, to shame the devil
              by telling truth: tell truth and shame the devil.
              If thou have power to raise him, bring him hither,
              And I'll be sworn I have power to shame him hence
              O, while you live, tell truth and shame the devil!

Master Wilburn Burchette answers Hotspur's skepticism in the brochure that sells his particular nostrum. Surpassing Glendower, Burchette says that not only can he call forth unearthly entities of inspiration, his music will allow the listener to gain these powers as well.

> We all know the power music has to control our emotions and intensify our feelings when utilized in the background of a motion picture or TV dramatization. Imagine then, what could be accomplished if a master musician and gifted mystic were to turn his full energies toward creating a mystical music which was specifically designed to be utilized as a tool in psychic practices and meditation. Ask yourself, what hidden psychic powers and energies you could call forth if you but had such a fantastic tool? . . . The possibilities are staggering![15]

The prerequisites for the creation of "serious meditation music" according to Burchette are a thorough knowledge of both science and art. Burchette also contends that "serious meditation music" can only be composed in a state of deep meditation, which contention presents obvious practical problems, not the least of which being the difficulty of writing notes on music paper with one's eyes closed.

Steven Halpern also believes that writing a "relaxation piece" requires that he "get into that state myself because it's a state-related experience." At the 1988 Music and Health Conference in Kentucky, Halpern explained that,

> Because music is a carrier wave for consciousness, if I'm in that state, that will get transmitted (which has been demonstrated by several interesting studies) onto tape, and then the listener will pick up on that. And it goes beyond just the notes themselves. So, I've had the situation where I've played some very nice music; I put it onto tape, but because my car had been hit in a parking lot on the way to the recording studio, even though the music sounded fine (I thought I had cleared that all out) . . . when I listened to it I found that it didn't work right. The notes sounded right; the impact wasn't there.[16]

Sometimes Halpern credits his body rhythms as shaping his compositional work: "I am playing my own nervous system. . . . I am playing my own biorhythms. . . . A fundamental principle is that the composer must compose him or herself. So, there is the Musician's Oath, the Pythagorean Oath, possibly parallel to the Hippocratic Oath, 'Physician, heal thyself.' "[17]

If this is true, then it needs to be asked why Halpern's body rhythms are particularly curative. Halpern has not established that his body functions in a particularly healthful manner, one that should be emulated by his listeners.

In fact, Halpern's fundamental principle of creating relaxing music, that the composer "composes himself," epitomizes reductionistic theorizing regarding the relationship between the composer and his music. Halpern is asserting that the listener shares the emotions involved in composing, that the composer's music is actually a "carrier wave" of his thoughts while composing. As the composer in the process of composition is primarily occupied with the act of composition, the listener to great music would be limited to mostly aesthetically meaningless technical considerations. Beethoven's thoughts during the composition of the opening to his Fifth Symphony, as is demonstrated by a study of the sketches, were primarily occupied with the correction of errors. Contrary to Halpern's theorizing, great composers attempt to eliminate from the audience's perception all traces of the compositional process, to create seamless music in which the listener remains ignorant of the composer and the arduous intellectual task that he underwent in order to create the composition. Beethoven rewrote the opening of his Fifth Symphony over fifty times to get it right. But the listener hears only the end product and cannot imagine Beethoven's Fifth beginning any other way than it does. Beethoven's audience responds with a panoply of intense and deep emotions blissfully ignorant of Beethoven's dissatisfactions with the first fifty versions.

There is yet another significant flaw in this concept: all listeners do not hear a piece of music in the same way. If one were to poll an audience of one thousand people listening to a Beethoven piano sonata and ask them to briefly describe their feelings, it is not unreasonable to expect that the result would show not 1 percent of the listeners in perfect agreement. Additionally, the emotional state of the listener produces a profound effect upon his interpretation of the piece. A person who has just experienced tremendous personal loss will very likely hear the Beethoven sonata in an extremely different way from a person who has recently experienced a joyous event. In the same way that a doctor cannot cure a crowd of one thousand people by entering a hall and administering a universal panacea, a music healer cannot claim to create an effective musical panacea for any group of listeners.

Halpern has taken the concept of state-specific music and turned it on its head. State-specific music refers to the state of the listener, not the music healer. Any practitioner must assess and treat each person as an individual. No doctor nor music healer can ethically administer any treatment without a feedback system that measures each individual's response to his or her treatment. When employing state-specific composition or improvisation techniques, the music healer must interact with the client if he intends to benefit him. Whatever Halpern composes in the sanctity of his home or recording studio may have beneficial, therapeutic effects for his listeners, as will any other piece of music by any other composer, but Halpern's claim for curative and relaxing properties cannot succeed until, and unless, he is willing to create music based upon his listeners' states of mind, and not his own. Paradoxically, since Halpern's modus operandi includes no interaction with his listeners, what Halpern is actually doing is performing therapy on himself through the creation of improvisational compositions based solely upon his own emotional state in front of an audience disenfranchised from the healing process.

Like Aeoliah, sometimes Halpern takes credit for his music, but at other times, such as in his book, *Tuning the Human Instrument,* Halpern gives credit to divine inspiration.[18] If this is the case, then it needs to be asked why celestial entities require Steven Halpern as a medium for their healing message.

Psychoanalytic and Transpersonal Hypotheses for Inspiration

"All the music ever written has been channeled," says Laeh Garfield in *Sound Medicine*.[19] Unfortunately, this statement does not address our desire to understand how music is created, for it neglects to answer two questions. If Beethoven merely channeled his music from some angel, where did the angel that dictated it learn *its* craft? And why is Beethoven's angel so superior a musician to Dittersdorf's angel?

In "Hearing and Inspiration in Music," Martin Nass explores the inspirational phase of music composition. "The composer's stance with respect to his experience of inspiration brings into focus issues of activity and passivity, and the issue of whether the source of inspiration is internal or external."[20] Brahms, like many other great composers, attributed his ideas as inspired by God. He even described a trancelike condition as necessary to his composing. Nass considered Brahms's self-abnegation as a "need to deny his own power or omnipotence."[21] Of Brahms's and other composers' trances, Nass writes,

> The shift to a more loosely organized state of consciousness is characteristic of the act of musical composition. As a consequence, there is the experience of ambiguity and confusion over the internal and the external. . . . His own impulses are thus *experienced* as external in origin and he becomes the copyist and not the creator. . . .
>
> A composer's denial of his own activity in inspiration involves the denial of his own aggression. The phenomenological experience of the self is defended against so that the composer will not feel its intensity while composing.[22] (emphasis added)

Whereas Nass suspects that the composer's tendency to defensively imagine that creation as "inspiration from outside" might be "a precondition for the progression of the creative drive to artistic creation,"[23] many composers have created beautiful music from an atheistic or agnostic philosophy, and many have denied inspiration. For every Brahms there is a Mussorgsky, for every deeply religious Salieri there is an insincere Mozart. Delius's imagery-invoking pastoral music was written by a man completely skeptical in regard to all theories supernatural, a philosophy that infuriated the deeply religious Fenby who transcribed so much of Delius's oeuvre once Delius became blind. Nass generously quotes Greenacre's 1963 work *The Quest for the Father,* subtitled, "A Study of the Darwin-Butler Controversy, as a Contribution to the Understanding of the Creative Individual." Greenacre believed that "if there is to be the fullest fruition of the creative force, there must be a coming to terms with and inner acceptance of the creative ability as belonging to the individual himself."[24]

If Brahms had a more philosophical bent, perhaps he would have wondered why God chose a rigorously trained classical musician like himself to compose great music, instead of just anyone who happened to have access to pen and paper, not to mention someone with a more pristine lifestyle (considering that Brahms was a frequent patron of houses of prostitution when he was not actually earning a living playing in them). If it was merely God writing Brahms's First Symphony, why did God have to struggle over it for twenty years after creating the universe in seven days?

Though Brahms might have believed he was divinely inspired he made no demand upon the listener to respect this belief as validating his composition. In fact, after playing the First Symphony on piano for the wife of his favorite composer, Robert Schumann, Clara Schumann made several suggestions on how to improve the work. Brahms followed her suggestions, throwing some doubt on the notion of a purely channeled work of music unless we are to believe that Brahms felt Clara Schumann knew more about music than God. It is evident that if Brahms felt God in some way responsible for his composition, it was not that Brahms considered himself nothing more than a copyist or channel. If he did, he would have ignored Clara Schumann's suggestions. Since he did not, we can infer that Brahms felt inspired to write great music, but understood that it was his personal responsibility to accomplish this.

When Palestrina wrote his great mass, now known as the *Palestrina Mass*, he claimed that it had been dictated to him by angels. Several hundred years later Daniel Dearing tells us that he is merely transcribing the music of extraterrestrials, while Aeoliah receives his instructions from Atlantis. Rosemary Brown, however, added another level—she received her compositions from defunct composers who, in turn, had received their music from God. The analogy to Palestrina breaks down when comparing the quality of his creations to the creations of Brown, Dearing, Aeoliah, et al. But whether Palestrina or Brown is writing the score, they share a common feature: a passage into an altered state of consciousness that is conducive to mystical thinking. The healthy composer's ego is strong enough to re-enter an ordinary, nonmystical state of consciousness; but for many, the prolonged visit into a more loosely organized mode of thinking carries a danger to the personal identity of the composer whereby he returns only partially, bringing with him mystical beliefs that become unhealthy and unrealistic in ordinary consciousness.

Surely no harm comes to Daniel Dearing as a result of his Pleiadian channeling while composing, but can the same be said for the "patients" of the New Age music healers who claim their divinely inspired music to have curative benefits? Personal delusions are offered as an alternative to medical science; and people who do not understand that Dearing is mistaken in his belief that the Pleiades star system harbors earthling-loving angels become prey to the delusional thinking of the self-professed music healer. It is tempting to say that those people foolish enough to believe the proffered fantasies of Atlantis and a paternalistic Pleiadian star system are undeserving of concern; but even granting credence to that cynical attitude, there are many music healers whose delusional systems are garbed in pseudoscientific jargon that gives the impression of a rational, scientific underpinning. The issue of culpability in the construction of these mystical systems of healing is not easily answered precisely because we cannot know, in most cases, the extent of the music healer/composer's own confusion between reality and fantasy, the extent to which the line between the two has been eroded by prolonged immersion in the altered state of consciousness.

Ken Wilber, a pioneer in transpersonal psychology (a branch of psychology stemming from the humanistic tradition begun by Abraham Maslow, which focuses upon altered states of consciousness) has begun studying the effects of the altered state of consciousness upon his and others' clients for whom they have prescribed daily meditation exercises. He found in his work that "distortions, pathologies or disorders" may occur in the beginning practitioner that require addressing by the therapist. A "psychic inflation," a "confusion of higher or transpersonal realms with the individual ego" can occur.[25]

In addition, one can never be sure when a composer writes about the process he employs for composition whether or not he is sincere, or, perhaps, using poetic metaphor to describe a process of creative thinking that has evaded successful description by musicians, philosophers, and poets.

The Art of Composing

Unlike the poet or novelist, the composer is confronted by an ineffably abstract task: the creation of a language. A novelist, for the most part, uses language to express his ideas about human interactions. The poet expresses his ideas regarding human interactions while simultaneously exploring the nature of language itself. The composer manipulates sounds, which are symbolic of nothing and represent nothing, but most do so in a way that communicates meaning to the listener. When a reader fails to understand a novelist's or poet's intention he may use a dictionary to uncover the meaning of a word; he may consult with other people who have read the same work to discover their interpretation, he may, perhaps, read the interpretation of readers from the past or present who have also puzzled over the meaning of the words. There are no analogous keys to understanding a musical composition. There is no expert, not even one who has studied a particular composer his entire life, that can offer anything more than a supposition in regard the most trivial musical detail. Musicologists who have devoted their lives to the study of Mozart cannot accomplish in a lifetime what the least trained proofreader can do in an afternoon's work. A misspelled word is quickly corrected in a writer's manuscript. But two hundred years after the composition of a piano sonata the experts are still arguing over whether Mozart intended a B natural or a B flat in a particular measure. An objection might be raised, how can we be sure what the poet or novelist intended? Can a book like *Ulysses* by James Joyce be understood in its entirety? Of course not, but there is enough correlation between Joyce's vocabulary and our own to allow the reader to comprehend those words not coined by Joyce, and, hence, to confer a meaning upon Joyce's writing that is not completely at odds with another's interpretation. An endless number of works could be written debating the meaning of *Ulysses* but not one sensible book can ever be written to explain what Mozart meant by the Piano Sonata K331.

In the opera *Mozart and Salieri* by Nicolai Rimsky-Korsakov, the author of the text, Pushkin, creates a fictional scenario in which this predicament is explored. Pushkin hypothesizes a vengeful and homicidal Salieri (Pushkin's story was later borrowed for the play *Amadeus* by Peter Shaffer) who desired to understand the method to Mozart's genius. Both composers wrote pieces for the same instruments using the same chords, and, frequently, even the same melodic fragments. Mozart was the greater composer: but why? Some might argue that Mozart is the greater because his musical structures were more complex, yet first, this does not explain why a Mozart piece written with a simple structure sounds better than a Salieri work with greater structural complexity. That also implies a pro-

gressive improvement in music, so that when a composer exceeds his predecessors in structural complexity the older music becomes obsolete,
which is obviously nonsense. Beethoven has not made Mozart obsolete.
No music theory has been developed that explains the difference between
Mozart and Salieri. None ever will, because just as the actual composition of music involves an ineffable process, so too does its appreciation.

The composer, therefore, is in an unenviable position of learning a
craft for which there is no right or wrong. He needs to study the past; all
great composers began by imitating works of their predecessors. However, a composer who repeats the past in his works is never considered
great. Though it takes a great amount of intelligence and musical ability
to write a four-part fugue in the style of Bach, the composer who does
only such imitative work can be assured that his music will never be
heard after he ceases to play it. So what is the difference between Mozart
and Salieri? Only this: one was Mozart and the other was Salieri.

To some, the lure of composition is as powerful and unforgiving as
the lure of the Sirens who enchanted mariners to sail toward their rocky
and fatal shore with music that Homer himself could not describe. Faced
with societal indifference and even disapproval, it should not be surprising that the composer, regardless of his talent, identifies with martyrs, or
heroes, or even aliens. That the composer is "abnormal" is undeniable and
that he is grandiose is certainly not shocking, but abnormality is not illness. Those theorists who attempt to understand composers by hypothesizing that their ability is intertwined with illness miss the boat. The great
composer communicates his brilliant message despite his abnormality,
not because of it. He is able to transcend his personal life so successfully
that his listeners will not comprehend his individual tragedy when he
chooses to deliver an opposite message. Mozart, Schubert, and Beethoven
were able to write music of astounding joy in the midst of personal
tragedy or deprivation. Stravinsky's happy little C Major Symphony was
written immediately following the loss of a most beloved member of his
family. Delius, who was cantankerous and cruel, even to his friends,

wrote primarily pastoral and gentle works. Conversely, Strauss, who had a charmed and bourgoise existence, could write the terrifying *Elektra* without ever having personally experienced a glimpse of the enormous tragedy he so successfully brought to life. Examples of such separation between the music and the lives of great composers are endless. It is rather the mediocre composer who is unable to express musically anything other than his own neuroses. Rossini, Schumann, and Smetana all reached points in their lives where their personal problems were so overpowering that they could no longer write effectively. Schumann's creativity was destroyed by his increasing madness. Those who attempt to equate Beethoven's greatness with his physical deterioration fail to account for the brilliance of an earlier work such as the Third Symphony in comparison to various later works of relative inferiority. This is not to say that Beethoven's late period is not, on the whole, greater than his middle period, but it should be remembered that his late period evinced the work of a more mature Beethoven, not a more diseased Beethoven.

In *Life Energy in Music* John Diamond writes:

And what of Beethoven with his obsession about Johanna? How much energy did that drain from him? How much hate did it engender in him? How much greater might he have been without that negativity? Perhaps he would have composed the Ninth Symphony some years earlier. And who knows what else he might have composed? Perhaps he would have lived longer and composed more.

In Berlioz's case it is easy to adopt the romantic notion that the idee fixe was a beautiful, poignant factor in his life. But was it so pleasant? What was the need that caused him to hold on to this idea with such fixity, with such obsession? . . . I believe that his life must have been severely impoverished if he needed to have these obsessions, in the same way the poor obsessed woman who was frightened of being raped must have led a very impoverished life to need to manufacture her delusion.[26]

Unlike Diamond, I cannot claim to accurately assess Berlioz's mental health at this late date. However, Diamond seems to infer that Berlioz's idee fixe was a symptom of mental illness. Whatever Berlioz's personal problems might have been, the idee fixe was, in fact, a musical technique of uniting four movements of a symphony in a way never before attempted, and its realization in the Symphonie *Fantastique* gave humanity one of the greatest symphonies of the nineteenth century. In addition, it served as the foundation for the musical structures of nearly all composers since that time, most importantly, Wagner, Liszt, and Strauss. Diamond's claim that Berlioz was "obsessed" implies a rigidity and repetitiousness in his thought processes that is the exact opposite of Berlioz's work. Berlioz is known, and rightly so, as the greatest innovator in musical history. Whereas Mozart and Beethoven and Brahms alter slightly the structures of their predecessors, Berlioz created entirely novel forms, including the tone poem, the orchestral song cycle, thematically unified symphonies, and the symphonic opera oratorio. He also explored areas of harmony and orchestration so advanced that another fifty years would pass before they were duplicated. This is not the hallmark of rigid thinking. Diamond also misunderstands the idee fixe in the assumption that Berlioz employed it in a rigid, repetitive manner. In fact, the idee fixe as used, for instance, in the Symphonie *Fantastique* is developed and modified during the course of the symphony's five exquisite movements.

In the first volume of *Life Energy in Music* Diamond writes:

From 1820 on, there is a change in Beethoven. There is now a complete absence of female friends in his immediate group. There is increased interest in prostitutes (whom he called "fortresses") and a great deal of what any psychiatrist would call latent homosexuality. This, in fact, may have been related to the jaundice which was first noticed at this time. Now in many cases of serious liver disease in males there is frequently a diminution of libido and an accentuation of female characteristics; for example, the penis and testicles may shrink in size and the breasts may enlarge. There may even appear on the skin what are called "spider naevi"—small blood vessels of the type of those of the uterus. All of this is in response to their elevated levels of female hormones. Every male produces female hormones which are normally broken down in the liver, but when liver activity is impaired, these hormones build up in the body, leading to an accentuation of female characteristics. It may be that Beethoven's great surge in creativity from this point until the end of his life, and with it the increased high level of the energy of his communications, is at least in part a result of his underlying sexual indecision (his kidney meridian problem) being "resolved" by the hormonal consequences of the liver impairment.[27]

Putting aside any objections to Diamond's hypothetical medical analysis of Beethoven's ailments and his theory of Beethoven being a latent homosexual stemming from his patronage of prostitutes, there really is no evidence of a "great surge in creativity" in Beethoven's life at this time. It is difficult to assess the meaning of purely subjective analyses of music. If Diamond means that he likes works from one period better than another, there is no difficulty. Personal preferences reveal nothing other than the personality of the assessor. Diagnosing mental states centuries after death may be fun, but unless supported by greater facts than personal opinion, nugatory. Diamond asserts that Beethoven could have created greater works had he not had his "energy drained from him" from his obsession with Johanna; yet he explicitly credits Beethoven's greatest creations as being the result of liver impairment. In reality, Beethoven complained about the draining of his energy in the *Heilige Dankesang* in the late A minor String Quartet. Diamond's contention that a lack of energy prevented Beethoven from writing great works when he was young and in love with Johanna is totally at odds with Diamond's other contention that Beethoven's liver disease promoted his writing of great works when he was older.

Some music healers have outdistanced Diamond's theorizing about composers' illnesses by contending that compositions created by physically or emotionally ill composers will actually contain the cure for their clients with these specific illnesses. Such a concept ignores several obvious defects, the first being, as in the case of Beethoven, that his music did not heal him; as no one can be closer to Beethoven's music than Beethoven himself, this apparent fly in the ointment should be adequate evidence for the inefficacy of illness-specific music. Secondly, the ailments from which Beethoven suffered were merely symptoms of a disease for which science has perfected a cure, in Beethoven's case, penicillin. Thirdly, most famous composers' illnesses were the result, in part, of the infamously poverty-stricken conditions under which they lived. Mozart might have lived to seventy years of age had he only had central heat and air conditioning. Finally, such a simplistic view of music as having illness-specific curative properties implies (1) that Beethoven's Ninth Symphony is irrelevant as a therapeutic tool for any client but those suffering from deafness or liver ailment caused by syphilis, (2) that a composer's works while healthy are analogously meaningless, and (3) that the music of a mediocre composer who suffers from some ailment is superior in its therapeutic value to the work of a composer who did not suffer from that ailment. Proclaiming music's illness specific curative properties also minimizes the real therapeutic value of music by ignoring its power as a tool for enlightenment, transcendence, and amelioration of various symptoms of illnesses.

In truth, great creative artists have managed to create great works of art regardless of their illnesses or (contrarily) perfect health. Mediocre artists, perfect health or not, create mediocre works.

Morality and Composition

In *The Secret Power of Music*, David Tame writes,

> Throughout the entire span of his adult life, however, Tchaikovsky was a man tormented. For he was a homosexual. Inwardly horrified with

himself and his tendencies, and embarrassed in the eyes of those who shared his secret, Tchaikovsky nevertheless failed to overcome his sexual inclinations. His homosexuality became the obsessive defect of his life. . . . Always nervous and highly strung, the composer found his life to be a ceaseless struggle against moral weakness and over-emotionalism. And it was a struggle from which, ultimately, he failed to emerge as victor.[28]

To accept Tame's propositions one must swallow his arguments whole. Homosexuality is horrifying, a tendency, a defect, and a moral weakness. It is also, apparently, defined in part by "over-emotionalism," which Tame does not define because he cannot. It must be assumed that composers who Tame likes are not overemotional. Such contentions are meaningless. They convey nothing but the author's likes and dislikes. Tame needs to conduct tests with music listeners to determine whether they can perceive sexual proclivities in a composer's compositions before simply asserting that homosexuality is a hindrance to successful musical creativity. There are many heterosexual composers who wish they had written Tchaikovsky's Fourth Symphony.

Tame writes,

If music patterns do hold a powerful sway over life pattern then Tchaikovsky's last three symphonies were a most inopportune manifestation for the composer to have left to posterity. There can be no doubt at all of the judgement which Confucius and his contemporaries would have passed upon these works. The basic philosophical theme of each of them is that which Tchaikovsky, in his letters and diaries, called "Fate." Each in their own way, the three symphonies tell the story of "Fate" and its relationship to the individual. Yet the individual is not so much abstract "man" as Tchaikovsky himself. And Tchaikovsky's "Fate" is not so much of a Universal Purpose or pre-ordained destiny as it is his personal subjection to the homosexuality which so tormented his conscience.[29]

On the contrary, there is plenty of doubt about Confucius's judgment. Tame assumes more than is defensible. Calling forth a dead philosopher to buttress his musical taste is no better than Rosemary Brown channeling Sir Donald Tovey to write a good review of her compositions. Tame concludes that,

> In Tchaikovsky's last three symphonies, we are called to move in another, and less enlightened, direction. What can, at least, be said of them is that they offer a most instructive lesson: that rarely, if ever, can the work of an artist rise above the main direction of his own consciousness. It is doubtful that a masterful music can ever result where the heart and mind of the musician are not themselves, for the main part, so mastered. Tchaikovsky the man was torn apart by the contradictions within himself: the spirit sought to soar; the flesh was fallow for the fall. Thus, while in music Tchaikovsky often brought forth beauty, he never attained the heights of true spirituality, and eventually, in his last symphonies, he became the instrument of the music of despair such as has proved to be the deadliest of plagues to numerous civilizations before our own.[30]

Setting aside the query as to what has set David Tame's homophobia all aflame, it is still amazing to read such a conclusion especially in the writing of Tame. Tame, after all, asserts that, "Wagner's motives in composing his music dramas were morally impeccable: to forge an art form which combined spiritual and deeply accomplished poetry with a music beautiful and sublime, all for the purposes of spiritually elevating the individual listener and bringing about enlightened social change."[31]

Wagner may be a better composer than Tchaikovsky; but, to infer, as Tame does, that an aesthetic judgement can be based upon the moral character of the composer requires us to suspend disbelief beyond the breaking point. Though it is difficult to defend my own hierarchy of moral righteousness in which I believe homosexuality is no moral crime, it nonetheless must surely strike the reader of Tame that his definition of moral impeccability, which places Wagner at the apex of right thinking and Tchaikovsky at its base, resembles nothing as much as it does the philosophy of Adolph Hitler. Tame condemns Tchaikovsky's music because he believes that Tchaikovsky's homosexuality is morally repugnant, and, contrarily, discovers in Wagner (a man of the most grotesque, anti-Semitic, and vilely racist opinions) a paragon of moral virtue. Such musical criticism we might expect in an alternate universe in which Hitler's minions succeeded in conquering the world and enforcing their own view of morality upon an enslaved populace, minus, of course, those homosexuals and Jews that they did, and would have, exterminated. But coming from a supposed New Age philosopher, Tame's criteria for moral righteousness are repulsive and frightening. Tame is not alone amongst music healers in his idolatry of Wagner and because so many music healers cannot separate the composer from his creation (a further extension of the belief that the composers' music is merely a reflection of his mental and physical state) they exhibit a few blind spots when it comes to studying Wagner the man.

Throughout his life Wagner unrepentingly espoused views of Aryan supremacy and the moral degeneracy of Jews, Orientals, and other "inferior" people. If his music did indeed reflect his malefic soul then we would naturally expect his audience to be restricted to like-minded neo-Nazis and white-robed Ku Klux Klan members. The fact that his music is loved and performed by Jews, homosexuals, blacks, Orientals, and others is the greatest proof for the contention that mental health and moral beliefs are in no way relevant to a composer's musical contributions. Wagner repeatedly espoused his hatred of whole races of peoples, his fervor most rabid when it came to Jews.

If emancipation from Judaism seems to us a prime necessity, we must test our strength for this war of liberation. We shall not gain this strength merely by an abstract definition of the situation, but by an intimate knowledge of the nature of our deep-seated, involuntary feeling of repugnance for Jewish nature. By this unconquerable feeling, what we hate in the Jewish character must be revealed to us, and when we know it we can take measures against it. By revealing him clearly, we may hope to wipe the demon from the field, where he has been able to thrive only under the protective cover of darkness, a darkness that we good-natured Humanists ourselves have offered him to make his appearance less disgusting.[32]

Cyril Scott was also impressed with Wagner's character. In *Music* he writes that Wagner "possessed one outstanding desire, namely the formation of a great brotherhood of art."[33] Scott neglects to mention that Jews would not be a part of this brotherhood. "This is very important," writes Wagner, "a race whose general appearance we cannot consider suitable for aesthetic purposes is by the same token incapable of any artistic presentation of its nature."[34] Scott describes Wagner as a "medium": "It was because Wagner possessed such a strong desire to help mankind that he earned the right to be used, even if only intermittently, by the Masters, Who recognised in him the finest musical medium They were likely to have for the next fifty years or so."[35]

Wagner would not likely have agreed with Scott's opinion that he was merely a channel. Wagner's ego was enormous, on par with that of Scriabin. Unlike Scriabin, who saw himself in the center of a relatively benign universe, Wagner thought himself surrounded by implacable swarthy foes. Scott attributes Wagner's strong opinions to a desperate struggle against "Dark Powers which work against the spiritual evolution of the race." These Dark Powers "were using every means at their disposal to thwart Wagner and his message."[36] Scott neglects to mention that Wagner identified the Dark Powers quite specifically as the Jews.

Deified by many music healers, Wagner did not himself entertain the idea of extraterrestrial inspiration for his own creations in his self-congratulatory essays, "On Poetry and Composition" and "On Opera Libretti and Composition." These are very mundane essays indeed; no angels, demons, or devas inhabit Wagner's musings. "The stock of attractive melodies has run out," he complains in "On Opera Libretti and Composition," "and without new ideas there cannot be much originality. Therefore I advise the composer of the latest style to keep a keen eye on his text, his plot and characters for inspiration."[37] It must be disconcerting to the scores of New Agers that Wagner never once credited Christ, Wotan, or any supernatural spirits for his awesome genius.

Not wanting to believe that the spirit world chose a narrow-minded, anti-Semitic, adulterous, narcissistic, beret-wearing Wagner to be their medium in the nineteenth century, New Agers often ignore Wagner's anti-Semitism, especially its role in the creation of his *Ring of the Nibelungen*. To see the gold-hungry gnomes with which Wagner peoples his lowest world as Wagner's portrait of Judaism is not simply conjecture. In 1848 Wagner wrote a fanciful history of the German people, titled "The Wibelungen: World History as Told in Saga"; this was his deluded view of German history, which formed the basis for the *Ring*. About Wuotan (Wotan in the *Ring*) Wagner writes, "The abstract highest god of the Germans, Wuotan, did not really need to yield place to the God of the Christians; he could be completely identified with him. . . . For in him was found a striking likeness to Christ himself, the Son of God. He too died, was mourned and avenged, as we still avenge Christ on the Jews of today." Later in this bizarre pamphlet Wagner puts in the mouth of Frederick the Great a fictional speech describing the rights of Germans to ownership of the Earth.

> In the German people there survives the oldest lawful race of kings in the whole world. This race issues from a son of God, called Christ by the remaining nations of the earth. . . . The Germans are the oldest nation, their king is . . . at their head [and] he claims world-rulership. There can therefore exist no right to any sort of possession or enjoyment, in the whole world, that does not emanate from him and require its hallowing by his sanction. All property not bestowed or sanctioned

by the Emperor is illegal, and counts as stolen, for the Emperor sanctions for the good, possession or enjoyment, of ALL, whereas the individual's gain is for itself and stolen from all. The Emperor grants these things to the Germans himself; all other nations must receive confirmation from their kings and princes as attorneys of the Emperor, from whom all earthly sovereignty originally flows, as the planets and their moons receive their radiance from the sun.[38]

Wagner's racial and personal narcissism infected the minds of future Germans less inclined to vent their madness in music. His world view, in which all land and property belonged first, foremost, and eternally to the German sovereign, became the goal of Adolph Hitler, who acknowledged his debt to Wagner's vision on numerous occasions. Remarkably, David Tame views Wagner as morally impeccable. "Wagner's reasons for composing in the first place, then, were entirely altruistic." Tame laments that "Wagner's motives (have not) been adhered to and emulated by the succeeding generation of composers. Wagner's innovations would have represented the climactic entrance into a new world of music—music of perhaps equal or even greater beauty than the music of the classical and romantic eras."[39]

In fact the opposite is true. Wagner's music did serve as a basis for a succeeding generation of composers as well as composers contemporary to Wagner. The symphonies of Bruckner, the tone poems and operas of Richard Strauss, the opera *Mephistofeles* by Boito, and the early works of Schoenberg are all clearly derived from Wagner. Schoenberg's *Die Gurrelieder* is thought by many to be the culmination and fruition of Wagner's musical ideal and Strauss's *Salome* and *Elektra* fully realize the vision of the music drama Wagner developed from his predecessor, Berlioz.

Tame admires Wagner's innovations, much of which may be traced to Wagner's lack of a thorough musical training when young. "In Wagner's later works," writes Tame, modulation occurred so frequently that no real sense of key survived. This was a fateful challenge to all thinking musicians, one of a magnitude which cannot be overestimated. Serious Western music had always been firmly grounded upon the concept of tonality, no matter how increasingly sophisticated the actual practice of tonality had become. Yet Wagner, in *Tristan and Isolde* and other works, had questioned the infringibility and inveteracy of the entire tradition. It was an overt questioning which could not be merely forgotten or ignored by the rest of the musical world, any more than Einstein's Theory of Relativity could have been bypassed by the scientific community.[40]

But the same is true for Berlioz before him, Beethoven before Berlioz, Mozart before Beethoven, and continues to be true today. Tame is blinded by his fetishistic idol worship of Wagner, as becomes abundantly clear when he tars Mussorgsky with the same brush and paint he uses to praise Wagner. Mussorgsky, he asserts,

was largely self-taught, and gave precious little heed to the established rules of harmony, etc. as practised and adhered to elsewhere during his day. A nineteenth-century musical Jack Kerouac, he composed freely according to the whims and dictates of his mental and emotional being. If a tonal phrase sounded right in his head, accurately expressing his own feelings, then he wrote it down, irrespective of any rules of key or harmony. . . . Much in the Jack Kerouac, beat-poet style, since Mussorgsky's art reflected a consciousness undisciplined by such notions as artistic correctness or spiritual motive, the result was often the naked portrayal of those less desirable levels of the human mind. Frequently, Mussorgsky's tone-sequences convey emotions which are very much of a downward direction—desolation, anguish and psychological pain. Mussorgsky was also one of the earliest composers to place so much emphasis on speech patterns in music—melodic sequences similar to the sounds produced when human beings ask a question, express a doubt, shout in anger or yelp with fear.[41]

Substituting the name Wagner for Mussorgsky in the paragraph above from Tame's book would ring just as true. Even Tame's characterization of Mussorgsky as a Jack Kerouac-like character is suitable for describing Wagner's own life. Tame complains that Mussorgsky depicted emotions of a downward direction—desolation, anguish, and psychological pain which we recognize as the hallmark feature of such tragic Wagnerian operas as *The Flying Dutchman* and *Tristan and Isolde.* Does Tame believe that Wagner's operas contain nothing but hebephrenic glee? Wagner wrote music dramas in which he explored the complete range of human emotions, as, of course, did Mussorgsky.

Mussorgsky's "emphasis on speech patterns in music" was nothing more than an adoption of Wagner's use of it, which Wagner championed loudly as one of his own self-proclaimed brilliant innovations. The freedom from classical tonality that Tame praises in Wagner's prelude to *Tristan and Isolde,* he condemns in the prelude to Mussorgsky's *Boris Godonov.*

Cyril Scott presents an opposing view of Tame's philosophy of music in his book *Music.* He remarks that some listeners of Mussorgsky's "spiritually educative music" may not

> realize the full significance from a spiritual-evolutionary point of view of thus portraying squalor and sordidness in music. If, however, we imagine for a moment the consciousness of the perfected Man, we must realise that one of the factors in that consciousness is the power to see beauty in everything. As he who can only love his friends and kindred has not acquired the true unconditional Love-consciousness expressed in the maxim, "Love thy neighbor as thyself," so he who can only perceive beauty in the *obviously* beautiful has not attained the *true* perception of Beauty. The soul that would evolve must evolve in all directions, and in order to reach the highest, must not shirk the lowers; he must, in the proverbial phrase, "go through hell to find heaven."[42]

Scott admired Mussorgsky's ability to depict deprivation in order to "arouse that hatred of bondage which resulted in the Revolution. To the more evolved soul, including that of the artist and the writer, he showed the beauty in squalor."[43] Mussorgsky's realism repulses and confuses Tame, who finds the composer's fealty to the bitter truth of the typical Russian's life too honest for even an enlightened individual's own good. Tame remarks pointedly that Mussorgsky's truth was not elevated and spiritual.

> For an artist to "portray truth" when that truth is secular, means no more than to express his own personality. Whereas Mussorgsky spoke deridingly about "varnish" and "tinsel trappings" in his portrayal of men, the idealists such as Handel and Beethoven had consciously avoided depicting the imperfect, mortal nature of people. To them, it was preferable to outpicture the divine spark within all men, which they hoped and believed that their music would itself help to nurture. It is within Mussorgsky's works that serious Western music descends from the plane of idealism and divinity to the level of human personality for virtually the first time.[44]

Not "virtually" the first time. In fact, Mozart's opera *Marriage of Figaro* was so free of gloss and idealization that Beethoven could not bear to credit Mozart with the vulgar creation. Beethoven found *Figaro, Don Giovanni,* and many other pieces immoral. Tame does not mention Mozart's immortal immoral vulgarities such as his choral canon "O Du Eselhafter Martin," which begins "O leck mich doch geschwind in Arsch," and proceeds in scatological humor to its conclusion. Jesse Helms, the Parents' Music Resource Center, and many other moral watchdog groups would be irate if they knew that the characters in *Cosi Fan Tutte* were indistinguishable from the vulgar adulterers represented in soap operas and talk shows daily.

In regard to Tame's two examples of Handel and Beethoven there are two flaws in his thinking: the first being that Handel "avoided depicting the imperfect, mortal nature of people." Handel did so repeatedly in his operatic works, which are, however, not frequently performed today, which may account for Tame's error in this regard. It is sometimes forgotten that Handel wrote more than the Hallelujah chorus from the *Messiah*. The second flaw is in assuming that music drama can be created without a foundation in the real world. Beethoven could not bring himself to cope with this problem and, hence, wrote no operas. His lone singspiel, *Fidelio*, though musically brilliant fails as music drama due, in part, to Beethoven's inability to create any tension by portraying Pizarro, the story's antagonist, as so unmitigatingly and inexplicably evil as to be laughable. Beethoven recognized his own failure and never attempted an operatic work again. The great operas of Western music invariably portray multifaceted human beings struggling with issues of morality. Tame seems also to have overlooked the complex issues of fealty and love so poignantly portrayed by Wagner in *Tristan and Isolde* and he is not critical of Wagner's human comedy *Die Meistersinger,* which is as secular as *Boris Godonov* and lacks *Boris*'s political punch, containing only a lame, chauvinistic finale glorifying a German king for no reason touched upon in the opera. Operas by Wagner or Mozart that do not fit Tame's hypothesis are not acknowledged. Not surprisingly, the only operatic work of Mozart that Tame does acknowledge is *The Magic Flute* about which he enthuses because of its "Masonic belief that art was an instrument which should be used for the elevation and freedom of humanity." Anyone familiar with *The Magic Flute* knows that the character that enchants every child, the character who has the most stage time and music, the character that most closely reflects the vital, vulgar, funny person that was Mozart is Papageno, who refuses the Masonic initiation and the pompous trappings of the esoteric Temple and is nevertheless blessed with the thing he wants most, a wife, who is his equal, Papagena. Mozart explicitly describes esoteric, secret societies as believing that all women are unworthy of trust, incapable of wisdom, and nothing more than chattel, the reward for proper behavior within the all-male fraternity.

An insurmountable obstacle in contending that *The Magic Flute* is an opera containing Mozart's glorification of Masonry is that though Mozart, an occasional Mason, wrote the music, he did not write the text. The libretto was written by Emanuel Schikaneder, who, two years prior to writing the libretto in 1789, was booted out of the Masons because of his wild and disrespectful behavior. He instructed Mozart to write the music for the Papageno character for Schikaneder himself. Thus, Schikanader, a deposed Mason, who wrote the text and assumed the role of Papageno, was able to mount the stage nightly and denounce the misogynistic Masons knowledgeably and unmercifully. The text abounds in sarcastic references and the opera ends with complete disclosure of a silly Masonic secret ritual.

Tame chooses to condemn composers who personally displease him with faults that he ignores in composers that he likes. Of Stravinsky he writes, "His long-standing poverty [did not] deter him from maintaining a whisky intake of the kind that would be expected to kill most men."[45] Nowhere does he condemn Beethoven, whose predilection for alcohol more than equalled Stravinsky's. Womanizing and adultery are two character defects to which Tame is blind and deaf; he never discusses Wagner's cruel, adulterous treachery, Beethoven's penchant for prostitutes, or Brahms's adulterous obsession with Clara Schumann and his own fealty to whoredom. If a composer Tame does not like has no known moral defects, he will go to great lengths to concoct one. Tame writes, "Debussy walked and moved about like a cat . . . he kept scores of cats as pets; he bought feline ornaments (and this, even when he was penniless and hungry) . . . he made a point of frequenting the Parisian rendezvous, Le Chat Noir; and the composer even conspired to be born a Leo."[46]

Poor Debussy, some New Agers have him busier before he was born and after his death than he was while living. According to Rosemary Brown he is now a painter; Tame thinks Debussy conspired to be born a Leo; and Cyril Scott claimed that Debussy visited Atlantis prior to being born. Ancient Egypt and mythic Greece were Debussy's own choices of imaginary peregrination. No great composer has yet set an opera or symphonic poem in the fabulous Atlantis, which, "as every occultist knows," in its inundation and destruction brought with its ruin the loss of "the scientific knowledge of the application and potency of Sound," which in itself "had wrought such havoc."[47]

Laeh Garfield reports that,

> All the music ever written has been channeled. . . . The realm of music has its own spiritual helpers and archangels, who sing tunefully to all those who concentrate their life's growth via music. Whether one is a secret composer basking in obscurity, a struggling artist who isn't able to sell the fruits of their labor, or a well-established luminary, the spirit helpers channel to all. Many catch the same message and interpret it in their own way. When this happens with the musically successful, several songs that are very much alike may appear on the charts . . . and, if the songs are timely by Universal standards, all can be hits at the same time.[48]

Garfield's presumption that all music is channeled from the higher planes is at least more democratic than the ideas of her brethren, who prefer to limit divine inspiration to those composers whose music they personally prefer. Tame wants his reader to believe that Wagner received his instructions from the Great White Brotherhood, whereas Mussorgsky could not get his foot past the door of the brotherhood's lodge. What one realizes, though, upon reading Tame, is that he likes the *Ring* and that he dislikes *Boris Godonov.* The beauty of Garfield's conception is that it allows us to imagine not just Brahms receiving aid from "spirit helpers" in the composition of his "Alto Rhapsody," but also the same for Robert Reed and James Avery as they penned the words and music to 2 Live Crew's hit rap song, "Bad Ass Bitch." If I were to believe in spirit guides, I would prefer Garfield's egalitarian vision, in which celestial beings can inspire such classic lyrics as "Me so horny, me so horny."

If the purpose of the New Age music healer/composer is to create musical works equal to or greater than Wagner's in the service of human spiritual evolution, it makes infinitely more sense for the self-proclaimed heirs of Wagner to hone their musical skills rather than devote so much energy to verbal justification and rationalization regarding their motivations and spiritual righteousness. Great music serves human spiritual evolution regardless of its composer's moral or spiritual defects; mediocre music is mediocre regardless of its composer's moral or spiritual correctness.

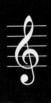

4. Systems: Right Concentration

A Mahatma and his wife came along, bringing a stringed instrument with them. They plucked at the string and began to sing a song.

As they began to sing, the Mahatma sang in one mode, his wife sang in another mode, and they played the instrument in a third mode.

And the Gosavi said, "Die, you miserable wretches!"

And they kept silent.

Then the Gosavi left.[1]

The Diatonic Chakra System

Most New Age music healers exhibit a remarkable and simplistic predilection for the Western classical music C-major scale. It is remarkable in that they apply this uniquely Western, tonal device to philosophies opposed to Western tradition, and it is simplistic because it ignores the fact that the C-major diatonic scale is but one of several scalar systems derived from Western music. The seven pitches of the C-major scale—C, D, E, F, G, A, and B—are but seven twelfths of the pitch material used in Western music, the other five pitches being D♭, E♭, G♭, A♭, and B♭. Over and over again we will find the New Age music healer who uses Eastern healing systems equating the seven diatonic pitches of C-major with the seven chakras of the body. Considering that Indian music has its own scale systems and predates Western society's invention of the C-major scale by several hundred years, it requires a monumental lack of respect for Indian culture to claim that sacred healing properties in the Indian tradition can only be realized using non-Indian music. I was not able to find a single music healer in any publication who ever associated the chakra system of healing with authentic Indian classical music.

In *Tuning the Human Instrument*, Steven Halpern explains that his Spectrum Meditation, in which the key of each movement is keyed to a color, is also scientifically keyed to the seven chakras which "recent research in psycho-acoustics" has verified.[2] The chakras are linked in ascending order from first to seventh with the ascending pitches of the European devised C-major scale: 1=C, 2=D, 3=E, 4=F, 5=G, 6=A, 7=B.

Halpern is the music healer most often credited for this simplistic system, but though Halpern claims that there is scientific research to substantiate his cross-cultural hybridization, this is unsupported by any documentation. There is no reason to link the seven chakra centers with the seven major tones of C, D, E, F, G, A, and B. Nor does Halpern even attempt to explain why the seven pitches of the C-major scale should serve as the basis for the chakra system he lifts from ancient Indian religion, as opposed to, for instance, the seven pitches of the B♭ melodic minor scale or the seven pitches of the F harmonic minor scale. There are some five hundred seven-pitch scales in Indian classical music (only one of which comes even close to the intervals of the Western C-major scale) to choose from in constructing a musically isomorphic system for chakra healing. Yet Halpern, who criticizes the concept of Western music as belonging to "dead, white, European men,"[3] nevertheless chooses a system of tonality devised by these dead, white, European men to define the music appropriate for his oriental philosophy of healing.

Don Campbell says that "our common scale [*sic*] . . . evolved" from "heaven," descending from Do, which equals God, the creator or *Dominus*, to Si for Siderial [*sic*], to La for Voie Lacte (the Milky Way), to Sol for Sol the Sun, to Fa for Fatus (Destiny), to Mi for Microcosmos, to Re for Regina Caeli (Queen of Heaven), to Do.[4]

Though Campbell credits this heaven-inspired attribution to an antique tradition, the truth is that this charming construct was built by Herbert Whone in his *Hidden Face of Music*, published first in 1974, which in turn reflects heavily the influence of Rudolf Steiner, who explained the derivation of the *solfège* syllables in 1914.[5] Equating the Western diatonic system with God reflects a nineteenth-century manifest destiny philosophy in which only white men are capable of appreciating spirituality, art, and science. One can almost hear the music healer condemning the twenty-two *sruti* system of classical Indian music as being nothing more than a heathen abomination.

In *The Secret Power of Music*,[6] David Tame asserts that the major scale is mirrored in the planetary conjunctions of five planets and the asteroids. Here again, a music healer finds justification for the European C-major scale in the heavens. For the two planets that Tame omits from his scale, no rationalization is offered. John Beaulieu claims that eight tuning forks pitched in the C-major scale are useful for healing. Incidentally, Beaulieu suggests tapping the tuning forks together, which is not a good idea if you want them to maintain their pitch and pureness of sound. Beaulieu believes also that, "When tapping the tuning forks our intention is important!" He believes that a listener can pick up the intentions of the tuning fork tapper from the sound of the fork. To support this belief he relates a personal anecdote about himself in which he falls asleep to the sound of a piano tuner tuning a piano. "I remember at one point the piano tuner striking middle C over and over. I must have heard him play it thirty or forty times. Then there was a period of silence for two to three minutes. I drifted off in the silence.

> Then out of the silence I heard middle C again. This time the note sent shivers up my spine. The sound was completely different and at the same time I knew the note was the same. Then I heard it again and again. It was like a concert—there was something very special about this middle C. I opened my eyes and to my surprise I saw the piano

tuner standing next to the piano. And sitting at the piano playing middle C was Rudolph Serkin.[7]

It is unclear how this anecdote supports Beaulieu's hypothesis about
intention being perceptible in tuning forks since even if the story is
accepted as true, and not illustrative hyperbole, both the piano tuner and
Serkin's intentions were identical, namely the testing of middle C for correct intonation. The story appears only to point out that Serkin's technique
is superior to the piano technician's despite the fact that they have the same
intention. Beaulieu's fascination with the repeated C has been brought to
life by Kay Gardner in her cassette tape, *Sounding the Inner Landscape.*[8]
Side one of Gardner's tape contains a seven-chakra meditation in which
the listener is asked to think healthy thoughts about the seven chakra centers, one at a time, while chanting in unison to Gardner's alto flute performance. Each of the seven musical interludes consists of the repetition of a
single tone, C in the first section, D in the second, to B in the last, thus rendering Halpern's major scale chakra system to its absolute minimal presentation. The choice of the C-major scale as the medium for Indian religious healing philosophy is, again, disrespectful. However, a listener able
to sit through twenty-six minutes of the C-major scale presented in
unprecedented slow motion, I admit must be in a meditative state, or dead.

Only the diatonic pitches of the C-major scale appear in William
David's "Integrative Processes" chart in his book, *The Harmonics of
Sound, Color, and Vibration.* He notes that these pitches correspond to
chants practiced by Tibetan monks.[9] However, Tibetan monks do not now,
nor have they ever chanted the diatonic C-major scale. And, I hazard, they
never will.

In *Music and the Elemental Psyche*, R. J. Stewart introduces the "ex-
panding spiral of music," his version of the circle of fifths; but he neglects
to include the chromatic pitches and instead creates a circle of fifths and
augmented fourths that have no relation to the natural harmonic series,
Eastern music, Western music, or any musical system known. Stewart fol-

lows this spurious circle of fifths with other "hermetic" inventions that account for only seven of the twelve pitches of the Western chromatic pitches, or less.[10] Stewart's circle is a meaningless placement of the seven diatonic pitches; a simulacrum of the true circle of fifths of Western musical practice. This is a puzzling non-utile construction equivalent to restating Einstein's famous formula $E=MC^2$ as $E=M$, creating a formula that is neither true, helpful, nor enlightening. There are certain scientific and musical theories which, when simplified, still yield beneficial insights. But Stewart's circle of "imperfect fifths" serves only to destroy any sense of meaning that is contained in the actual circle of fifths.[11]

In his *Harmonies of Heaven and Earth*, Joscelyn Godwin lists numerous seven-tone C-major-scale philosophies, but does not imply that one or more of these make any particular sense. Godwin has done his research, and his lists are actually a useful compendium for one interested in the various and sundry nonfunctional hermetic theories of the last two millennia. However, Godwin also falls into error when he equates Indian *sruti* with the diatonic C-major scale, as in his rendering of a British version of a thirteenth-century Indian music theorist's work on animal-tone correspondences. Godwin should have been aware of the fact that ethnomusicology is a relatively new field and early British practitioners of it regularly adulterated foreign music, rhythms, and pitches to fit European taste; in this instance they were oblivious to the subtleties of the twenty-two *sruti* system. Early British ethnomusicologists were more interested in "correcting" Indian music than accurately representing it.

Harmonies of Heaven and Earth is thorough but flawed. Many of Godwin's facts are simply not so, and some are based on faulty research, as exemplified in his reliance on nonscientists in regard to music's effects on plants. In addition, Godwin finds favor in certain of his collected hermetic theories that are no more sensible than those he brands as spurious. Godwin's grasp of ethnomusicology and astronomy is equally tenuous, and he occasionally lapses into enjoyable, though stertorous, sermons on hellfire and damnation.

Once the devil has souls in his grip, seduced maybe by songs of love and ease, they are condemned to a Hell where the perversion of harmony into horrendous cacophony is relieved only by the hopeless and still more horrible silence of its frozen depths. . . . The Devil's musical skill serves one purpose only: the seduction of souls. He inverts the purpose of God-given harmony, using the power of music to drag the soul not up but down. It was from fear of this that the Fathers and Doctors of the Church mistrusted all music that was unsanctified by a sacred text—a fact which held up for centuries the development of instrumental music—and the exoterically-minded Mullahs of Islam invoked the Prophet Muhammad's authority for an absolute (and always unsuccessful) ban on all music whatever.[12]

Godwin's hectoring Christianity does not distract from enjoying his tome. It adds a mordant and intriguing touch. Godwin rails against popular music, declaring it immoral and dangerous. Rock music, he says, "propels its feelers—one cannot say its listeners—into a trance-like participation which is a perverted image of the higher modes of listening."[13] Godwin's primary objection to rock music is its capacity to transport the listener—I cannot say the feeler—into a "trance-like" state, the very aim of many music healers.

Music healers, though their music may be more related to popular Western music such as rock than they care to admit, often clothe their music in oriental symbolism. The Hindu chakra system is a ubiquitous presence in their writings. Halpern draws upon the "scientific" testing of the chakras as support for his music theories. So do Drury, Garfield, McClellan, Gardner, Hamel, and Beaulieu, to name but a few who have not only drawn on this Eastern concept but have also, in typical Western fashion, chosen to systematize it.

"The soul is located in the heart chakra," Shirley MacLaine explained to Larry King and his television audience on September 10, 1985.[14] We Westerners, it seems, cannot be satisfied with the ambiguous nature of Eastern ideas, and in our anxiety over the very essence of ineffable doc-

Table 1
Chakra-Pitch Congruencies

Chakra	McClellan	Halpern	Garfield	Watson and Drury	Gardner	Aeoliah
1st	A	C	Boogie-woogie hard rock heavy metal Bob Dylan	Paul Horn Herbie Mann Philip Glass Brian Eno	C, C♯	C
2nd	E	D	Reggae	Brian Eno Pink Floyd	C♯, D	D
3rd	A	E	Reggae	Manuel Gottschung Klaus Schulze	E	E
4th	C♯	F		Brian Eno	F, F♯	F
5th	E	G	Joan Baez	Aeoliah Brian Eno Ligeti	G, G♯	G
6th	G	A			A	A
7th	A	B	New Age music soft jazz	A♯, B	B	
8th					All sound	

trine rush to distort and compartmentalize it. Kay Gardner is so dissatisfied with the ancient tradition of chakras that she decided to improve upon it by adding an eighth chakra to the millennia-old seven. All of the above-mentioned authors have decided that the Indians are just not vigorous enough in their application of chakras and mantras and so have created their own Western-style congruency charts so that there need no longer be any question as to what is appropriate for each chakra. In my Western way I list their Chakra-pitch congruencies in Table 1.

In *The Healing Forces of Music*, Randall McClellan lists a chart of chakra-pitch congruencies identical to that of Halpern (and Halpern's followers), but includes a coherent list of objections to Halpern's concept.

McClellan points out that the major scale is a European invention, "whereas the concept of *chakras* comes from Hindu and Buddhist teachings. Eastern scales employ tuning systems that are very different from our own." Regarding the Halpern ordering, McClellan objects to Halpern's "proposition that we all resonate to the same pitches." McClellan believes that every individual resonates at his or her own frequency. McClellan also finds the correspondence of the seven chakras to the C-major scale "entirely too simplistic, too convenient, and I think, a bit capricious because chanting mantras to tones was done long before the invention of our equal tempered scale."[15]

McClellan's objections include some dubious ones. His eighth objection is, "The fourth and seventh scale degrees of our major scale cannot be derived from the harmonic series,"[16] a statement that is no more true for the fourth and seventh than it is for the second, third, and sixth. McClellan's belief that humans have any resonant pitch also fails to ring true. But overall his reasoning in regard to the absurdity of assigning the seven chakras corresponding pitches in the key of C is unusually sound. Disappointingly, McClellan's flirtation with logic is brief, as he follows his list of objections with his own approved list of chakra rhythmic chants, approved because he found them to be "particularly attractive."[17] Whether or not they are attractive, they are all in simple triple time (six/four or nine/four), which ignores the traditional Indian penchant for duple and septuple meters.

Kay Gardner and other recent practitioners have taken the assigned pitches for each of the seven energy centers of the body (chakras) and have created short compositions that use the assigned pitch as the tonic or key note. For example, in music for the first energy center, the composition is in the key of C-major, for the second it is in the key of D-major. Music for the third energy center is in E-major; for the fourth, F-major; the fifth, G-major; the sixth, A-major, and, finally, B-major is utilized for the crown of the head. The historical justification and a clear theoretical basis for this practice remains obscure, however, and physical benefits have not been tested and published.[18]

McClellan's rebuke of Halpern, Gardner, et al. includes the accurate report of music healers' collective failure to test and research their claims. Steven Halpern has claimed to have demonstrated the validity of his healing system repeatedly and with literally thousands of people. In a lecture at the 1988 Music and Health Conference at Eastern Kentucky University, Halpern responded to his critics, explaining the origin and validity of his chakra healing system:

> Where it came from is something that has been around for thousands of years. I was the first person to put a sound track to it. But people like Sir Isaac Newton, Sir Francis Bacon and many other traditions for thousands of years have talked about chakras. Many have talked about the colors that people see with them. Many people have talked about the tone. But they hadn't actually composed music for them. Some people can actually look at a chakra and see a color. . . . I asked in my research . . . could [you] feel color, feel a sound? And they said, "Well, you hear it in your ear; you don't feel a sound." So this testing was, "If you COULD feel it, tell me where you feel this sound." Then they said, "Well, this is funny but I feel C around here, G around here, and F's around here," and statistically we found that, sure enough, that was one of the main paradigms that exist in the literature. Now, there's literature on that. There are references for that in my book. There's also literature on that that disagrees.[19]

Granted, Sir Isaac Newton, and Sir Francis Bacon never talked about chakras, but Halpern's status as the progenitor of the chakra-based diatonic music healing field allows him some leeway in regard to the facts. Halpern and his colleagues do not stop at pitch/chakra relationships, of course, but draw up myriad congruencies in which the seven chakras are assigned specific colors, body parts, ailments, vowel sounds, and so on.

The Colors of the Chakra System

After building up a hunger for systematization with an Indian appetizer, the music healer is ready for the main course, the pitch/color congruencies. Halpern's chakras of the C-major scale are assigned correspondent colors, specifically red, orange, yellow, green, blue, indigo, and violet in ascending order.[20] However, Halpern's westernization of pitches and colors does not escape the wrath of his brethren. Steven Halpern, Barbara Ann Scarantino, and William David hew to C-major and ignore the chromatic pitches. Cousto determines color-pitch congruencies by equating spectral frequency to sonic frequency. Laurel Keyes's color-pitch correspondence "came" to her "through Roger Stevens, musical instructor and member of the Los Angeles Symphony, and from a book printed in the last century." She acknowledges that, "Sound and color are not produced in the same way. Few people will agree on which key corresponds to which color. They have received some intuitive impressions about it, which may be correct for them, but I prefer the ordered logical sequence of . . . the prismatic pattern."[21] Keyes and the majority of music healers pick red for the tone of C, but even if there is a congruence of pitch and spectrum, it is unclear why C is so often chosen as the corresponding tone to the lowest visible frequency. Why not choose the tone A?

Nevill Drury explains his difficulty with Halpern's system of C-major scale/chakra-pitch congruencies by saying, "It does not match the vibratory colors actually used by practitioners of Kundalini Yoga. It also has the drawback of imposing a framework which is not based on the actual belief system itself."[22] Drury's criticism that Halpern's ordering of pitches and colors fails to correlate is at odds with that of the Halpern supporter who argues that, "Halpern's system is symbolically appealing to the extent that the base chakras of *mulakhara* and *svadisthana* correlate with the dynamic segments of the spectrum and the energy levels progress musically to the more transcendent reaches of consciousness associated with *ajna* and *sahasrara* and the meditative colours of indigo and violet."[23] This supporter of Halpern, who is diametrically opposed to Drury, is as knowledgeable about chakra systems as Drury, because he *is* Drury. Finding himself both in utter disagreement *and* complete agreement with Halpern's pitch-color congruencies, Drury and co-author Andrew Watson discover the happy medium of mutual fuzziness by stating that the "problem with Halpern's system, however, is that the colours do not equate with the traditional symbolic colours ascribed by the Hindus themselves to these chakras. Nevertheless, the point is made that one can progress meditatively from the active energy levels to the more introspective realms of spiritual awareness using these musical scales."[24] Agreeing, disagreeing, and somewhat agreeing and disagreeing with Halpern, Drury eschews the creation of a seven-pitch scale/chakra congruency system in favor of surgically separating the chakra/body-part relationships into twelve groups (rather than seven), and applies this surgically altered chakra/body relationship to the twelve pitches of the Western chromatic scale.

Drury's respect for Indian tradition is suspect in light of his suggestions regarding what music is appropriate for each chakra. Selecting a mostly homogeneous group of white European male composers to relate the meaning of the Indian chakras, Drury and Watson list over a hundred music recordings as appropriate, of which only two are by Indians.[25] (One is a Rajneesh Foundation recording which is not traditional Indian music. The other is a pop Indian recording by Chaifanya Hari Derter.) Not even one token Ravi Shankar record. Not even a Beatles tune with sitar. Drury and Watson's complaint about Halpern's lack of fidelity to the Asian source of the chakra healing system pales in comparison to the Western orientation of their music listening list.

In *Music Power,* Barbara Ann Scarantino amazes the knowledgeable reader by declaring, "In 1797, composer Andre Gretry published a list of musical keys, their psychological characterizations, and color vibrations as perceived by composers Rimsky-Korsakov and Alexander Scriabin, respectively."[26] Gretry could only have accomplished this feat had he the powers of precognition, as he died before either Scriabin or Rimsky-Korsakov were born. One could hardly expect more, but Scarantino then writes of Gretry's precognitive list, "These keys comprise all the twelve tones of the chromatic scale,"[27] which statement precedes her compilation of but ten of the twelve tones of the chromatic scale. There is still more. Scarantino's promised "color vibrations as perceived by composers Rimsky-Korskov and Alexander Scriabin," are incomplete and erroneous. She attributes to them both the error of considering colors for a diatonic scale only, in G-major, neglecting five other pitches. Scriabin did not neglect D♭, one of his favorite keys. "All pieces of music," Scarantino foolishly asserts, "are written in a specific key, but the key is not always designated in the song's title, except in some classical pieces (Vivaldi's Concerto in D-major, for example)."[28] Considering that Scarantino discusses Scriabin, she should have known that many pieces even by her avatar were written in no specific or even discernible key. It is also difficult to excuse her apparent ignorance of Stravinsky, Schoenberg, Strauss, Bartok, et al. In a listing of recommended classical music pieces, Scarantino names: "Chopin's 'Polonaise,' " " 'Midsummer Night's Dream,' " " 'Evening Star' by Wagner," and "the Parsifal music by Wagner."[29] That Scarantino is not familiar with the pieces she suggests, but is merely parroting Corinne Heline, is evident in the misapplied titles she offers in her list. The "Parsifal music" is obviously an awkward rendering of the prelude to *Parsifal*, as discussed by the more musically literate Heline. I do not believe that by "the Parsifal music" Scarantino means the entirety of the five-hour music drama. "Chopin's 'Polonaise,' " is as utile a clue as saying "Mozart's Symphony," and " 'Midsummer Night's Dream' " is even less helpful than "the Parsifal music by Wagner."

To understand what Scarantino is parroting, one must read Corinne Heline, the religiose matriarch of the New Age pseudoscience of color and music. About Heline, whose work has served as the foundation for many color-music schemes, Steven Halpern notes, "Although she never says where she gets her information, Ms. Heline traveled in some well-respected esoteric circles. Reading what she has to say about the relationships between sound and color and astrological signs and seasons opened up broad new vistas for me. . . . I can pinpoint some inconsistencies in her systems, but the overall gestalt is one of inspirational information and love."[30] Heline drew upon the eccentric work of Scriabin for her scheme of color-coordinated music. However, Scriabin was too precise for her to adapt his specific scheme to her own vague, grandiose ideas. Refraining from analyzing each movement from Beethoven's nine symphonies, or the principal key of each symphony, she chose to group all nine symphonies together as "blue, indigo, violet, purple, and amethyst," a color they share with (according to Heline) the entirety of Wagner's *Ring, Parsifal, Lohengrin,* and all the "Masses and Gospels set to music by various composers."[31] As Heline makes no mention of any of Beethoven's other works, it can be assumed that all of Beethoven's music is a shade of purple.

Part of Heline's confusion regarding pitch-color equivalencies no doubt lies in her confusion regarding optics. Chapter 2 of *Color and Music in the New Age* opens, "Goethe, who was, perhaps, the world's most profound color-scientist." The line presages bewildering claptrap such as "purple, like peach-blossom, is not found in the Newtonian spectrum." Heline confuses the area of color or hues with the simple, natural reality of the normal solar spectrum; and "peach-blossom," (depending on the peach) is found in the 600- to 640-millimicron wavelength of the solar spectrum.[32] Heline also puts forth the remarkable claim that there are "presently invisible to the average physical eye" many colors which only certain people "who possess ability to explore inner realms" may see. For those of us who do not possess the requisite abilities, understanding is impossible because these invisible colors are "too exquisite for description."[33] It would be easy to test this fanciful assertion, simply by marking pieces of paper with illustrations visible only in the infrared or ultraviolet frequencies and asking possessors of this special talent to describe them. Heline's misunderstanding of the physical capabilities of human beings is gross and her condescension palpable and smug. She credits "Nicholas Roevich, possibly the foremost artist of our time by reason of his high spiritual attainment" with employing "previously unknown astral colors in his magnificent creations."[34] By this, perhaps, she means purple and peach-blossom. It must be that those of us who do not see in Roevich's art any value are not spiritually enlightened enough.

The story of the emperor's new clothes is a most apt analogy for Heline's claim that certain enlightened individuals today can see colors that the unenlightened cannot. There are similarly music healers who claim to be capable of hearing frequencies beyond normal human capacity. Such claims can be easily tested.

The principal human object of Heline's worship is not Roevich, but Richard Wagner. Of her books, all but one invoke the Bible or Christ, or link healing and music in their titles; the one exception is *Esoteric Music—Based on the Musical Seership of Richard Wagner*. To invoke Wagner in a book on music healing is not a crime, but to think Wagner spiritually enlightened is criminally unenlightened. Wagner's character has always been a difficulty, especially for those who love his music. Heline is either ignorant of Wagner's noxious personality or disagrees with the near unanimous appraisal of Wagner's diseased personality ("near unanimous," because Nazis and their ilk consider Wagner's character pristine). Heline wrote that Wagner was extremely sensitive to the influence of color, noting that the composer wore nothing but silk "next to his body." By this, I assume she meant to say that he wore silk underwear. Wagner's decision to let nothing come between him and his silk was "not just an eccentricity," Heline reassures. "It was a case of a nervous system which had become responsive to color's subtle radiation beyond the ordinary range of human sensitivity."[35] Wagner's ordinary range of human sensitivity is unfortunately evident in his "Judaism in Music" from *Stories and Essays*. "So here we reach the starting point of our enquiry: the revulsion aroused in us by Jewishness. The Jew will never be excited by a mutual exchange of feelings . . . but only by matters of particular egotistic interest to his vanity or to his sense of profit. This makes him to our ears more ridiculous than sympathetic."[36]

Wagner indeed believed his own evil words regarding sympathy when he lashed out at the prematurely deceased Felix Mendelssohn.

> He showed us that a Jew can possess the greatest talents, the finest and most varied culture, the highest and most delicate sense of honour, and that none of these qualities can help him even once to move us to the depths of our being as we expect to be moved by art, and as we are when one of our own great [Aryan] artists simply opens his mouth to speak to us. It can be left to technical critics, who have probably reached the same conclusions as we have, to confirm, by reference to Mendelssohn's music, the undoubted truth of our remarks.[37]

Perhaps Corinne Heline unconsciously saw herself as one of these technical critics when she wrote, "Felix Mendelssohn was perhaps the only one of the celebrated composers who did not know the whiplash of poverty. He was born into a family of affluence and was reared amid serene and congenial surroundings. . . . Those composers whose works show forth the undying beauty of spirit—for in that their immortality consists—acquired their great mastery through lifetimes of sorrow and toil."[38]

At least Heline does not attribute Mendelssohn's failure, in her opinion, to "show forth the undying beauty of spirit" to his being Jewish, as did her idol, Wagner. Heline claims Mendelssohn's color note to be pink, as it accords with that "of his personal life since he was truly privileged to view life through rose-colored glasses."[39]

"The color notes of this great music-seer, Richard Wagner," gushes Heline, "shine forth in a soft cast of mauve-purple together with a glittering radiance of white and gold."[40] All of Wagner's colors are represented in Heline's list of "Color Significance of the Twelve Zodiacal Signs." Pink is nowhere. In Heline's explanation of "The Spectrum and the Human Aura," Wagner's mauve-purple color note denotes "purification and transmutation of the personality into spirituality" Pink is absent. Wagner's colors cure numerous and sundry ailments in Heline's "Scientific Application of Color." Pink does not appear, even as a token homeopathic treatment for pink-eye. Pink does not even garner a mention in her "tonal equivalents of form and color."[41]

It is interesting to note Heline's omission of Jewish composers and musicians in all of her works, with the exception of Mendelssohn, who did not actually practice Judaism, to whom she assigns the only color with no healing or spiritual properties.

While there is no direct evidence of anti-Semitism in Heline's *Color and Music in the New Age,* her hysterical and heretical Catholicism is ubiquitous, and sometimes unintentionally comical. "The truth shall make you free" is how she ends her chapter "Color Therapy," an admonition implying that those who find her theories absurd are not Christian enough. Before Christ, Heline wants us to know, man was practically blind and deaf. "In the time of Homer, about 900 B.C., humanity had become conscious of three colors: red, orange, and yellow."[42] Of course Homer might object to this characterization, Homer who wrote of "ear splitting Dionysus" that "his dark hair was beautiful, it blew all around him, and over his shoulders, the strong shoulders, he held a purple cloak."[43] Purple, again, that color which Newton, in Heline's clouded vision, forgot. "Not until the Golden Age of Greece was lovely green clearly perceived. The higher more spiritual colors became visible at a much later date. This was not until man had developed certain spiritual faculties which enabled him to study spiritual laws,"[44] Heline explains.

In the hopes that humankind has evolved spiritually, and that we are able to view the colors of the spectrum, I offer Table 2, a list of music healers' color-pitch congruencies.

Without a doubt the music healer with the most comprehensive systematization is Kay Gardner. Her "Chart of Color, Sound and Energy Correspondence" has a 1984 copyright and was revised in 1987[45] (see Figure 1). The title is not nearly comprehensive enough. Gardner notes correspondence between colors, musical pitches (chromatic scale), vowels, spinal contacts, chakras (energy "wheels"), color-transmitting, endo-

Table 2: Color-Pitch Congruencies

Pitch	Scriabin	Drury	McClellan (Absorb)	Gardner (Transmit)	Gardner Schwarz, Manners, Scarantino	Halpern	Cousto	David	Heline	Keyes	Aeoliah (Color)	Aeoliah (Higher Octave Color)
C	Red	Red	Green	Red	Turquoise	Red	—	Red	Purple	Red	Red	White
C♯	Violet	Red-Orange	Turquoise	Red	Turquoise	—	Blue-Green, Blue	Red	Red	Red-Orange		
D	Yellow	Orange	Blue	Orange	Electric Blue	Orange	Blue	Green	Yellow	Orange	Red-Orange	Violet
D♯	Glint of Steel	Amber	Indigo	—	—	—	—	—	Yellow	Orange-Yellow		
E	Pearly Blue, Shimmer of Moonlight	Yellow	Dark Violet	Yellow	Lavender	Yellow	—	Yellow	Red	Yellow	Orange-Yellow	Ruby-Violet, Gold
F	Dark Red	Green-Yellow	Darker Violet	Yellow	Lavender	Green	Red, Red-Violet	Purple-Violet	Blue	Yellow-Green	Green	Pink
F♯	Bright Blue	Green	Ultra-Violet	Green	Rose	—	—	—	Violet	Green		
G	Rosy Orange	Blue-Green	Red	Sky Blue	Peach	Blue	Orange-Red	Orange	Black, White	Green-Blue	Sky Blue	Electric Cobalt, Royal Blue
G♯	Purple	Blue	Red-Orange	Sky Blue	Peach	—	Orange-Red	—	Green	Blue		
A	Green	Indigo	Orange	Indigo	Moon Golden	Indigo	Orange, Orange-Red	Indigo	Electric Blue	Blue-Violet	Indigo	Emerald Green
A♯	Glint of Steel	Violet	Yellow	Violet	Pale Yellow	—	Yellow-Orange	—	Gold	Violet		
B	Soft Blue	Magenta	Lemon	Violet	Pale Yellow	Violet	—	Blue	Misty Blue	Red-Violet	Ultra-Violet, Rainbow	Golden Yellow

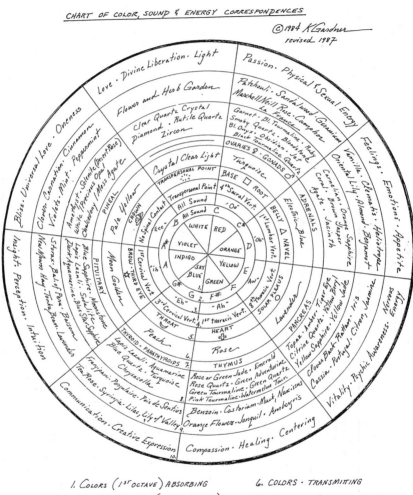

CHART OF COLOR, SOUND & ENERGY CORRESPONDENCES

© 1984 K Gardner
revised 1987

1. COLORS (1ST OCTAVE) ABSORBING
2. MUSICAL PITCHES (CHROMATIC SCALE)
3. VOWELS
4. SPINAL CONTACTS
5. CHAKRAS (ENERGY "WHEELS")

6. COLORS · TRANSMITTING
7. ENDOCRINE GLANDS
8. GEMSTONES
9. PURE ESSENSES
10. ESOTERIC ATTRIBUTES

crine glands, gemstones, "pure essences," and esoteric attributes. Nor is this a simple list of single attributes. For instance, under the color green Gardner notes, "Rose or Green Jade, Emerald, Rose Quartz, Green Adventurine, Green Tourmaline, Green Quartz, Pink Tourmaline, and Watermelon Tourmaline," as the congruent "gemstones."

Gardner seems ambivalent about her pitches. All the attributes are clearly delineated. There are no blurred boundaries, but the chromatic pitches slop all over. Maybe this can be accounted for by the fact that Gardner divides her pie into eight slices, whereas there are twelve chromatic pitches. The note C is just over the border of white in red; D is in the middle of orange; E is likewise clearly contained by yellow. White, however, entertains no pitches, but separates B and C with "All sound." F straddles yellow and green, decisively indecisive; and G♯, A, and A♯ all share indigo; but the prize pitch, the pitch nonpareil, is D♯ (or E♭). Even after revising her chart in 1987, Kay Gardner neglected E♭. Did no one, between 1984 and 1987 inform Gardner of this omission, or was E♭, the key of Beethoven's *Eroica* Symphony and *Emperor* Concerto, too aggressive, too masculine, too bold to take its place amongst the eight "Turquoise, Electric Blue, Lavender, Rose, Peach, Moon Golden, Pale Yellow, and Crystal Clear light" transmitting colors of the sixth category? Could Gardner not conceive of a "pure essence" for E♭? "Clover Bark, Rattan, Iris, Cassia, Portugal, Citron, and Jasmine" serve for Gardner's E. Could not garlic, oregano, curry, hot pepper, steel, blood, and phlegm serve for E♭? There is even room for an endocrine gland (seventh category), as Gardner left out the islands of Langerhans, which in light of the fact that Napoleon, the original dedicatee of the *Eroica*, was exiled to the Isle of Elba, seems eminently suitable. As for the tenth category, esoteric attributes, in which E is represented by "vitality, psychic awareness, and nervous energy," could not E♭ be represented by boorishness, overbearing machismo, logic, and that feeling of bloatedness one develops after eating too much?

Unlike many of her colleagues, Gardner offers no list of zodiacal-

Table 3
Zodiac-Pitch Congruencies

Pitch	Drury/ Halpern	Scarantino	Schneider/ Godwin	Schneider (earlier)	Heline	Steiner*
C	Aries	Virgo	Cancer	Aries	Virgo	Aries
C♯	Taurus	Aries	Capricorn	Cancer	Aries	Scorpio
D	Gemini	Libra	Libra	Libra	Libra	Gemini
D♯	Cancer	Taurus	Aries	Capricorn	Taurus	Capricorn
E	Leo	Scorpio	Taurus	Taurus	Scorpio	Leo
F	Virgo	Sagittarius	Leo	Leo	Sagittarius	Pisces
F♯	Libra	Gemini	Aquarius	Scorpio	Gemini	Libra
G	Scorpio	Capricorn	Scorpio	Aquarius	Capricorn	Taurus
G♯	Sagittarius	Cancer	Sagittarius	Gemini	Cancer	Sagittarius
A	Capricorn	Aquarius	Virgo	Virgo	Aquarius	Cancer
A♯	Aquarius	Leo	Gemini	Sagittarius	Leo	Aquarius
B	Pisces	Pisces	Pisces	Pisces	Pisces	Virgo

*Steiner designates these congruencies "Key-Zodiac"

pitch congruencies. She may have kept finding herself one short on pitches (due to the absence of E♭) and given up. The twelve signs of the Western zodiac are irresistible, however, to most music healers. A table of various music healers' zodiac-pitch congruencies is shown in Table 3.

In *Healing and Regeneration Through Music*, Corinne Heline writes "Every musical genius . . . realizes his greatest achievements in composition in the key which governs his life."[46] In the book Heline claims that Beethoven's key was C♯. It may be argued that the C♯-minor String Quartet is Beethoven's greatest work and the *Moonlight* Sonata may be his best known piano sonata. It could be argued with just as much validity that Beethoven's key note is C, the key of the Fifth Symphony, or D, the key of the Ninth, or B♭ for the *Grosse Fuge*. In fact, C♯ is less easy to defend as Beethoven's key than almost any other due to the small number of works he wrote in C♯. Beethoven, Heline claims was a "Martian" in the astrological sense. On the other hand, she claims "Uranus . . . came in Wagner not only to awaken, but to sweep man, body, soul, and spirit into the Cosmic Consciousness."[47] It cannot be discerned in Heline's writing (with some exceptions, such as Beethoven's C♯ key note) what key notes governed the lives of which composers. Heline tells us that Bach was a Mercurian and says, therefore, that his key note is that of the planet Mercury, and that Wagner's key note is based upon the tone of Uranus, but whatever pitch Heline ascribes to these and other composers is as trivial and pointless as the C♯ she ascribes to Beethoven. Of course, many composers have favored keys and will compose in them more frequently than in others. Sometimes this is just a matter of practicality, as in eighteenth- and nineteenth-century symphonies that employ French horns or trumpets. Since these instruments were equipped to play only certain pitches in certain keys, writing a symphony in F♯-minor would have proven impractical, as no such instrument as the F♯ horn (actually, an F♯ crook) existed at the time. Symphonies in F♯ became feasible after the invention and adoption of the valved (chromatic) horn in the mid-nineteenth century. There are, in addition, many more reasons composers select certain keys for certain pieces. Mozart wrote four horn concerti, three of which are in E♭, and not because E♭ was Mozart's key note.

The Sound of the Universe

Perhaps Shirley MacLaine, another New Age matriarch, was actually channeling the late Corinne Heline when on the Larry King television show of September 17, 1987, she reported that Galileo said "All the planets revolved around the moon."[48] When music healers apply their scientific skills to astronomy, they report that the celestial bodies have specific pitches (see Table 4).

Table 4
Celestial Body–Pitch Congruencies

Pitch	Drury	Scarantino	Stewart	Cousto	Campbell	Schneider/ Godwin	Tame
C	Mars	Sun	Moon	Sun	God	Mars	6th moon of year
C#	Venus			Earth, Pluto		Moon	7th moon of year
D	Mercury	Moon	Mercury	Mercury, Mars, Saturn	Moon	Venus	8th moon of year
D#	Moon						9th moon of year
E	Sun	Mercury	Venus		Earth	Venus	10th moon of year
F	Mercury	Venus	Sun		Planets	Sun	11th moon of year
F#	Venus			Jupiter			12th moon of year
G	Mars	Mars	Mars		Sun	Saturn	1st moon of year
G#	Jupiter			Uranus		Mercury	2d moon of year
A	Saturn	Jupiter	Jupiter	Venus, Neptune, Moon (syn.)	Milky Way	Jupiter	3d moon of year
A#	Saturn			Moon (sid.)			4th moon of year
B	Jupiter	Saturn	Saturn		Galaxies		5th moon of year

Hans Cousto's *Cosmic Octave* is a nonpareil work of pseudoscience that explores the "origin of harmony" as derived from the current estimates of planetary distances from the sun. Cousto's grand scheme is the revitalization of the poetically charming but scientifically outdated notion of a harmony of the spheres. Pythagoras attempted to justify the musical customs of his peers by relating the tetrachordal Greek modes to the orbits of the heavenly bodies. Pythagoras neatly accounted for the intervals using the astronomical knowledge of his time. But Pythagoras's ex post facto rationalizations for the music of his time were built upon a view of the solar system that we now know is completely wrong. Pythagoras's calculations, therefore, have been rendered meaningless in regard planetary relationships to intervals since Copernicus corrected our view of the solar system.

Those who wish to resurrect Pythagoras's view of a solar system in perfect harmony with music are failing to recognize two disqualifying factors: (1) Pythagoras calculated orbits in a geocentric universe, a model we now know as false, and (2) Pythagoras's planets were believed to exist in perfectly fixed spheres, as opposed to the imperfect and frequently changing ovoid orbits in which the planets actually travel. Cousto's attempts to validate part of Pythagoras's ideas by showing how the universe occasionally can be described as having qualities not completely contradicted by Pythagoras as "proof" that he was on the right track utterly disregard and place in disesteem the entirety of Pythagoras's philosophy. Pythagoras was not attempting merely to validate human belief systems, but rather to ascribe universal properties to a fixed and logical scientific model.

The music Pythagoras was attempting to rationalize (not mythologize) was the music of ancient Greece, not the music of modern Western cultures. Thus, applying Pythagoras's musical theories to today's Western musical practice is as culturally and logically meaningless as assigning chakras to the diatonic C-major scale.

Cousto is valiantly, if misguidedly, trying to "save the phenomena" of the ancient harmony of the spheres by using contemporary astronomical data to give his theories a cloak of scientific verisimilitude. Fortunately for the lecherous reader, Cousto's ramblings on the motions of planetary bodies orbit around Tantric sexual notions and chakras. He illustrates the concept of a tuning fork with a drawing of "A Tantric Scene," in which a man and a woman engage in sexual intercourse.[49] This illustration of sexual intercourse in a treatise on acoustics must surely be a first.

For the most part, tables and charts preoccupy Cousto. He calculates planetary orbits and rotational periods corresponding to pitches by dividing numbers in half until he reaches a number corresponding to a frequency in hertz in the middle register of the piano. This is an anserine assignation, as arbitrary as equating the number of ducks in the state of Pennsylvania on a given day, say, 901,120 ducks, to the pitch A. If you divide 901,120 enough times you do reach 440, a frequency for A above middle C. But, you may argue, the number of ducks fluctuates too much to calculate a proper Pennsylvania duck-to-pitch correspondence. You would be right. The number of ducks undergoes flux, and the orbits of the planets do, too; and any measurement of a distance is good only for a particular moment. Pluto, for instance, is now (at the time this sentence was written) the eighth most distant planet from the sun, but more often it is the ninth.

Cousto spices up his dry mathematical correspondences with occasional advice on sexual matters and the like.

"You can only have ecstatic sex when your excretory organs are functioning well. . . If there's a feeling of pressure on the bladder, you won't be able to let go when you make love. . . . It is not only important to concentrate on your sexual energies to get more out of sex, you must also make sure that your bowels and bladder are in good shape."[50] Cousto's chart depicting the seven chakras, unlike such bland, sexless representations in books like Halpern's *Tuning the Human Instrument,* which show a simple body shape outline, is of a comely, long-haired lass with a strand of dark hair playfully curving around one of her breasts. The depiction of the *Muladhar* chakra is very special indeed.[51] "Music composed in G is . . . very stimulating and is therefore not recommended for Roman Catholic priests."[52] I assume the admonition applies to nuns as well. Puccini was obviously unaware of it in the composition of his *Suor Angelica,* an opera that takes place completely within the confines of a nunnery, and whose tonal center is G. Perhaps Puccini was making a bold and ironic commentary on the nature of gravid Sister Angelica's dilemma.

Like Corinne Heline, Cousto is an advocate of pitch and color therapy. After explaining that the "color of an earth day . . . corresponds to the

65th octave of an earth day . . . from orange-red to red," Cousto shows the significance of the color "orange-red" for life: "The color orange-red has a direct influence on the process of cell division. In Canada, for example, Professor Max Luscher proved in several series of experiments that the growth of testes in drakes can be controlled by the use of color. . . . The testes of drakes reared beneath an orange-red light grew twice as fast as those of drakes kept below pale blue light."[53]

Cousto's Tantric philosophy luminates the pages of his tome in bright primary colors, whereas Heline's is painted in the pastel hues of theosophy steeped in Roman Catholicism. Cousto roars that the "Immaculate Conception is nothing more than the suppression of sexuality on a godly level" in a typical misunderstanding of that dogma as describing the conception of Jesus as sexless rather than sinless.[54] Heline would have her reader know that, "The Bible will be the supreme textbook of life to the very end of his [man's] evolution on this planet. Not until the conclusion of this great incarnational cycle will he fully comprehend the meaning of the biblical promise, 'Ye shall know the truth, and the truth shall make you free.' "[55] Presaging other New Age preachers, Heline sees no problem in combining disparate religious philosophies.

Joscelyn Godwin compiles an impressive and comprehensive list of hermetic zodiac-music system "mysteries." His imaginative "Anthroposophical Table of Correspondences" includes zodiacal signs, senses (such as smell, taste, ego, thinking, and warmth), body parts, consonants, and powers. Godwin's table has a curious lacunae in his category of "Power," however, in that five zodiacal signs are assigned no attributes. Godwin does not explain this gap, but it is apparent that there are five missing attributes because the original correspondences were constructed over a diatonic scale that misses five chromatic tones.

When perusing various hermetic systems it is a good idea to keep in mind how frequently esoteric music theorists find themselves in a bind trying to reconcile the numbers twelve and seven. Whenever one comes across a theory obviously lacking in five constituent parts, it is likely that one is looking at a system borrowed from an earlier inventor who was only concerned with the seven pitches of the diatonic scale. Clumsy adaptations account for the obvious gaps.

Striking similarities abound in different music healers' pitch-zodiac correspondences. Drury's and Halpern's tables are identical to Steiner's but only for the pitches C, D, E, F♯, G♯, and A♯. A transposition of an augmented fourth makes up for the difference in those six pitches. Evidently, Drury and Halpern are basing their system on Steiner's, though they fail to credit him. Scarantino cribs Heline's rendering, briefly abandoning her usual source for correspondences: Halpern. Marius Schneider's earlier correspondence is clearly derived from Steiner, beginning with a minor third transposition and proceeding in drops of minor thirds from the initial Aries. Heline's zodiacal table is simply a reiteration of the correspondences of Max Heindel, who decided that the five black keys of the piano must represent the five first signs of the zodiac. Heindel assigned major keys and their relative minors to the signs, but Heline simplified this so that each sign of the zodiac is represented by the tonic pitch of the major key selected by Heindel.[56]

In *Music for Inner Space* Nevill Drury devotes the majority of his esoteric analysis of music to the Tarot, and whereas he is eager, in *Healing Music,* the book he cowrote with Andrew Watson, to draw relationships between the Indian chakra system of healing and Western music, nowhere does he make a connection between Indian *srutis* and the twenty-two Greater Arcana cards in the Tarot. This is a pity, aesthetically, because there are twenty-two *srutis.* Jack Schwarz devotes the majority of his book *Human Energy Systems* to the Tarot. He lists the Greater Arcana and a pitch, color, sign of the zodiac, and planet for each card. As is to be expected, problems arise when one tries to squeeze twenty-two Tarot cards into twelve pitches, the twelve signs of the zodiac, and the celestial bodies. Some of Schwarz's cards have no zodiacal counterpart, but all have a planet, which creates problems. For instance, Jupiter, the planet, is given more than one pitch and one card. It shares colors as well. Schwarz gives

Mercury a pitch of B, but lists this frequency as both 493.9 cps and 466.1 cps while simultaneously listing A as 466.1. Accepting his rather inordinately high choice of a frequency for A if one must, there is still no possible way to interpret his other frequency of 493.9 for A, as this higher frequency will sound a major second above the lower, obviously no minor discrepancy. This is the first time I have encountered the intervallic distance of a major second (A to B) interpreted as the same as the unison.[57]

Schwarz, with his complex lists of correspondences and Drury, with his attention to the chakra system of healing, overlook the obvious: relating the twenty-two Greater Arcana of the Tarot system to the twenty-two *sruti* Indian tonal system, an oversight that allows Indian music theorists and fortune tellers both to breathe a sigh of relief. I can only hope that pointing out this trivial and coincidental numerical relationship does not engender yet another inapposite New Age intermarriage of disparate cultures.

Schwarz's *Human Energy Systems,* although not as comprehensive as Gardner's, is the most elaborate and detailed system of correspondences I reviewed. But his attention to the zodiac is not nearly as devoted as that found in the books *Life Streams* and *The Healing Energies of Music.*

The most prolific contributor to zodiacal interpretations of music is Hal Lingerman, whose *Life Streams* is nothing less than a day-by-day list of music one should listen to during the year based upon some rather superficial astrological and theosophical knowledge. Even astrologers would be aghast at the simplistic rationales that Lingerman uses for choosing music. The music he suggests for January 4 is Josef Suk's "Ripening." Suk was born on January 4. January 9 is for the music of John Knowles Paine, who was born on January 9. January 11 is for Christian Sinding, born on January 11. January 13 is Richard Addinsell, January 20 is Guillaume Lekeu, and so on and so on, all for the same reason. It is fairly easy to adopt Lingerman's plan without buying his book, because most unimaginative FM classical radio station programmers do exactly this, play a piece of music by a composer on his birthday.[58] Following this unhelpful listing of 366 days (Rossini was born on February

29 and Lingerman suggests Rossini's sonatas for strings for that day, which is most unfair to the piece because the day is so rare), Lingerman offers a table of composer's birth dates. Besides the 250-odd composers he lists are these strange additions: Walt Whitman, Gandhi, Vladimir Horowitz, Ignace Paderewski, Isaac Stern, Pablo Casals, and Rod McKuen. I can accept that Rod McKuen has written music, but is his "Balloon Concerto" really "a twentieth century masterpiece," as Lingerman describes it? And do McKuen, Sri Chimnoy, Cyril Scott, Martin Kalmanoff, and two dozen mediocre (at best) composers deserve inclusion whereas Stravinsky, Schoenberg, Bartok, Leoncavallo, Massenet, Boito, and Messiaen do not? The objection is subjective, admittedly, but Lingerman is offering himself as an arbiter of classical music listening, and his choices are worse than execrable.

In *The Healing Energies of Music* Lingerman evaluates composers in relation to their astrological signs (only their sun signs, actually). His failure to include Bartok in *Life Streams* is made clear by his comment, "Bartok's music is often strange and impersonal. . . . I have not found it to be therapeutic or renewing."[59] Disliking Stravinsky, Bartok, and Schoenberg does not disqualify Lingerman from publicly commenting upon his musical preferences; but his critical judgment is severely myopic. One would expect at least one of the three principal composers of the twentieth century to please.

In his "A Gallery of Great Composers," Lingerman makes some rather jejune comments on the greatest composers of the last five centuries, and he reveals a profound lack of knowledge about classical music in general. For Mendelssohn ("Aquarius-Air") he finds the frantic *Italian* Symphony "good for calming tense and agitated patients."[60] Perhaps Lingerman meant Mendelssohn's *Scottish* Symphony, which could have been on side B of his recording. "I find ('Aquarius-Air') Mozart's music uniquely different in quality and essence from other composers! It is somewhat pulsive, mysterious, at times will-o-wisp."[61] Of course Mozart's music is uniquely different from other composers, just as other composers are uniquely different from each other, but the curious attribution here is to the mysteriousness of Mozart, a quality in direct contradiction to the open honesty that best characterizes his works. About Franz Schubert ("Aquarius-Air") Lingerman lists his "main works" as including "Ave Maria; the nine symphonies."[62] I assume that by nine symphonies Lingerman means to include as companion to the *Unfinished* Symphony, the *Unbegun* Symphony, as Schubert wrote only eight symphonies. About Frederick Delius ("Aquarius-Air") Lingerman notes that "Delius's music is filled with the atmosphere of nature."[63] Regarding Delius, the author's observation is as illuminating as noting that water is wet. One might expect Lingerman to describe Beethoven as powerful, and, of course, he does.

In an extensive appendix Lingerman lists music appropriate for different seasons, by which he means that spring is represented by such works as Beethoven's "Spring Sonata," Britten's "Spring Symphony," Delius's "On Hearing the First Cuckoo in Spring," and so on. Lingerman lists Debussy's "Printemps" under summer, perhaps because he does not understand French.[64]

Whereas Lingerman uses simplistic astrology to create a system of music healing, David Tame uses a flawed understanding of astronomy to create his theory. He cites "Bode's Law" (by which he means the "Bode-Titius Rule," first enunciated by Johann Titius in the eighteenth century) as demonstrating that the planets of our solar system occupy orbits of perfect octave distance from each other. He ignores the distance of Mercury from the sun (an important omission necessitated by the fact that if the sun, the true center of the solar system, were used in Tame's figuring, the results would be even less defensible). One of Tame's tables depicts the "units of distance from Mercury" of the planets (and the asteroid belt). Using the distance between Mercury and Venus as equal to "1," he follows with obviously inaccurate ratios representing the distances Mercury to earth, Mars, asteroids, Jupiter, Saturn, Uranus, Neptune, and Pluto.[65]

Tame also concocts a table of "actual mean distances" that are meant to bolster credence in the applicability of the Bode-Titius Rule, but his "actual mean distances" are fantasy. At least Cousto accurately reports the figures for the average mean orbitary distances in his reformulation of the harmony of the spheres (and Cousto's illustrations are more memorable). In Tame's imagination all the planets are the same "pitch," with the exception of Neptune, which he would consider a perfect fifth above Uranus. He arrives at this unfortunately unexciting conclusion in which there is *no* harmony of the spheres, as all the planets are the same pitch (excepting Neptune), by equating the two-to-one difference in distance between each successive planet with the two-to-one difference between any pitch and its octave. Assigning the pitch C to Mercury, the planets according to Tame are pitched: C, C, C, C, C (asteroids), C, C, C, G, C (Pluto). But Tame is also dissatisfied with a celestial octave system, and one page after he endorses it he abandons it in favor of a planetary-pitch correlation based on the speed of the orbits around the sun rather than distances between the planets.[66] Tame arbitrarily divides a table of years into eight parts to reflect the diatonic C-major scale rather than twenty-two parts for the Indian *sruti* system, twelve parts for the chromatic scale, or five parts for the pentatonic scale. In any case, the revolutionary periods he lists are so inaccurate that further criticism of Tame's planetary-pitch systems is superfluous. In astronomical argot, Tame completely fails to "save the phenomenon."

R. J. Stewart, in the opening chapter of his *Music and the Elemental Psyche,* is one of the few New Age music theorists to abstain altogether from allotting colors or zodiac signs or planetary measurements to the pitches. As noted earlier, Stewart eschews the chromatic intervals in his esoteric theories on sound and healing. In fact, his frequent use of systems and charts seem incongruous in light of his disesteem for the Western penchant for systematization and classification. Stewart's first chapter, "Music and Changing Consciousness," is in large part a perseverative attack on "systems" and Western thought.

> The fallacy of authoritative systems, or even worse, occult and elitist systems, is our unfortunately conceptual inheritance from an orthodox

dogmatic male-dominated religion . . . but in this context we are concerned with its corruption of the power of music and magic in human consciousness.

Many esoteric works are elitist and dogmatic, even those claiming to carry us beyond the formal Church. . . . Most of these books are written by men and occasionally women—who were heavily conditioned by the orthodox Church . . . and in the case of writers prior to the twentieth century were often members of the priesthood. Within this false ambience of "authority," maintained by force of arms where necessary, is the image of the patriarch, an all-wise domineering male who utters "truths" that are "definitive."[67]

After thoroughly and coherently condemning the practice of systematization as being antithetical to New Age philosophy, Stewart seems to suffer from a sudden attack of amnesia, and with the same vigor with which he denounced systematization in chapter 1 he proceeds to report on, construct, and defend systems through the rest of his book.

The formal maps in our diagrams, such as the *Tree of Life* or the *Fourfold Elemental System* appear to be constant or even rigid to the superficial examination, but once they are enlivened by deeper imaginative attention, vital changes occur within their living matrices.[68]

and:

The non-systems [*sic*] illustrated should help us to rid ourselves of the false limitations of musical authority.[69]

and:

The systems are open-ended; they are fluid, accommodating, flexible. They are not rigid or authoritarian; you will not fail in any way if you do not follow them precisely.[70]

and:

> The diagrams are made as simple and direct as possible and may be
> used in several different ways. They are not intended to improve upon
> the remarkable . . . correspondences found in earlier works.[71]

And so on and so on. Stewart even creates a list of reasons, properly enu-
merated, to explain why he used his systems for explaining phenomena
that are not properly served by systems,[72] creating therein a system of systems in defense of phenomena not properly served by systems. I am
tempted to believe that Stewart's entire first chapter is some Swiftian self-
parody but Stewart's tone and ratiocinations belie such an ironic conclusion. I believe Stewart sees himself as a skeptical and pessimistic voice
of reason within the music healing field. His book often warns of a present, and even continuing, malaise in the field caused by unwarranted
optimism. "Far from suggesting that we are about to swing into a musical new age, I suspect that future generations . . . will see the twentieth
and twenty-first centuries as the nadir in the devolution of music within
human consciousness."[73]

Stewart sees artistic history in a way completely opposite to that of
Corinne Heline. He believes that music (and all the arts) have become
corrupted by civilization. Stewart's golden age of the arts is constantly
receding into the past, and he condemns the classical music that Heline
views as the peak of musical perfection. "The classical period of eighteenth and nineteenth Century music . . . extends into the twentieth Century. Although long-standing intellectual traditions are apparent in formal
art music, it nevertheless degenerates into a rigid set of entities frozen
upon paper by the notation system. The traditions become traditions of
style, even of pretension, rather than areas of shared consciousness and
experience."[74]

Referring to commercial popular music, Stewart writes that it is superficially trivial, but inwardly potent. It can be a most effective tool for shaping individual and group response. . . . Those with affirmed interest in "better forms" of music . . . find themselves tapping their feet to a loud radio playing in the street or humming a crude melodic phrase overheard from a television commercial.

Paradoxically it is at this gross and trivial level that we find the magical power of music, as opposed to the much lauded individual creativity of the serious composer which is not expressed to society at large. . . .

Due to lamentable ignorance and willful miseducation, Westerners think that they have no inherent magical music in their culture, and that all "magic" comes from the individual composer, often in the working out of his or her emotional crises. As we shall discover, there is an enduring and effective set of Western traditions for music that changes consciousness; this teaching has survived from the most distant past right into the present day, and it still works.[75]

Fairy Music

Stewart's pessimistic view thus excludes nearly all forms of music as vehicles for music healing. Classical music was too systematized; today's contemporary art music even more so; popular music Stewart finds himself tapping his feet to, but wishing he wasn't; and the jingles of television commercials, though hypnotic, fall short of the magical content he deems necessary for the purpose of music healing. Stunning as the revelation will appear, Stewart believes that the music best suited for the New Age has been handed down to us by elves. "Traditionally such [potent] music was transferred by individual tuition, sometimes between humans and Otherworld tutors, as in the fairy music taught in Celtic countries. We shall return to some of the ancient concepts in our later chapters, for they are not mere superstition but are a simple expression of musical power inherent in nature—both human and non-human."[76]

Stewart's belief in the participation of real fairies in the dissemination of music is not without its precedents. He says, "The elementals have been the subject not only of folklore but also of serious research, and present-day occultists hold a sophisticated view of them."[77] Stewart supports his statement with the results of research carried out by Ernst Hagemann in experiments by clairvoyants. Upon

> applying their second sight to the surfaces of gramophone records, they found them thronged with elemental forms—all dead. Looking through a magnifying glass, they could see even more of them! These, they said, are the lifeless replicas of the elementals who were constellated in the air, entered the microphone, and were "shadowed" upon the record matrix during the original live performance. In order to carry over these dead copies into the physical world via the reproducing device, one needs the cooperation of other, living elementals—tiny Gnomes, to be precise—whom the clairvoyants were able to perceive in the diamond or sapphire stylus. (One recalls that gemstones are traditionally associated with these earthy spirits.) Through the Gnomes' agency, the very same kinds of elementals—presumably Sylphs and Undines—could be seen emerging from the loudspeakers as had originally been captured in the recording process.[78]

"Unhealthy Music"

Tipper Gore, the wife of Vice President Albert Gore, was a cofounder of the Parent's Music Resource Center, an organization that attracted considerable media attention as it fought to be the arbiter of music selection for America's youth in the way that the Hay's Office controlled the American movie industry for the middle decades of this century. Gore's PMRC is active primarily in the field of popular music, where it has linked the music of rock 'n' roll artists with various societal ills. Regarding the impact of rock 'n' roll on teen suicide, Gore remarked in a 1988 interview, "I don't know that it is having an impact on teen suicide. . . . It's a delicate point very easily misconstrued for somebody to say, oh, she's saying that rock music or a song is going to cause a suicide. That's way too simplistic. I tried to make the point in the story about Sandy Hanson ... whose 14 year old son did commit suicide. ... It turned out that he was listening to a 'Suicidal Tendencies' album over and over. ... There were songs about suicide on that album."[79]

Today, rap is one of the leading contenders for musical bad boy. In the 1960s the Beatles and the Rolling Stones were considered to be demonic influences upon impressionable teenagers. Today, those profligate tunes accompany shoppers in supermarkets. A decade before the evil Fab Four, Elvis's gyrating hips scandalized a God-fearing nation. In the nineteenth century the German pun on the waltz craze labeled this new form of entertainment for the young "dirty dancing," and over two thousand years ago the newest music and dance crazes in Greece prompted its philosophers to bemoan the dissolution of Hellenic youth. In an odd alliance with the despairing mothers and fathers of today, music healers in our decade more often than not take Tipper Gore's side in the age-old struggle to prevent adolescents from choosing the music they wish to dance to at their parties.

Steven Halpern, considered the originator of New Age music, has made his attacks upon rock music an integral part of his music-healing philosophy. In *Tuning the Human Instrument,* he states that bone conduction is in part responsible for rock's sexuality. He reports,

> Electric bass players, for instance, knew intuitively what their groupie feedback confirmed: when their bass was powerfully amplified, these low frequencies "felt good"—especially in that place where the thighs meet the inverse vector of the torso. Unfortunately ... the very thing that was getting people aroused leaves them limp, due to the egregious assault on the sensitive nerve-endings and organs throughout the body. It's not just the ears that take a beating! ... An increasing number of rock stars, former paragons of virility, are reporting problems in that area.[80]

Halpern is being discreet when he does not identify what "that area" is, and he is irresponsible in regard to his fabricated claim that an "increasing number of rock stars" are becoming impotent due to electric bass riffs. Halpern continues his attack on rock 'n' roll (and other genres of music) when he describes his music-healing philosophy. He believes that the body is a "self-healing organism which chooses health when given the opportunity," but that a person can be "so addicted to certain rhythms that are counter to the natural heartbeat (such as some of the rock and disco rhythms we've heard before, heavy metal or break dance rhythms) that you are switched, and generally are choosing that which is not natural for the body."[81]

In the book he wrote with Louis Savary, *Sound Health*, Halpern and Savary clarify what these "certain rhythms" are. The authors report that, "One of the problems with much of rock and pop music is its standard rhythm, what is called the 'stopped-anapestic rhythm'—a 'short-short-long-pause' pattern. This stopped-anapestic rhythm tends to confuse the body and weaken the muscles."[82]

It is odd that anyone would take such an assertion seriously, yet the consensus in music-healing circles is undeniably clear. Halpern often cites his colleague John Diamond's theories regarding rock music's negative influences on the body. In 1979 Diamond wrote in his book *Behavioral Kinesiology*,

> Using hundreds of subjects, I found that listening to rock music frequently causes all the muscles in the body to go weak . . . [and] every major muscle of the body relates to an organ. This means that all the organs in our body are being affected by a large proportion of the popular music to which we are exposed each day. . . . Some groups and singers that tend to weaken our muscles are the Doors, the Band, Janis Joplin, Queen, America, Alice Cooper, Bachman-Turner Overdrive, and Led Zeppelin. In contrast, the Beatles never do.[83]

Diamond and Halpern/Savary are in agreement in their belief that the "anapestic beat" is what causes rock music's ill effects upon the body. But, this "anapestic" rhythm is not exclusively associated with rock 'n' roll, nor with jazz or the blues, as Halpern/Savary and Diamond imply. It is a very common occurrence in classical music as well. The Bauern-Marsch in Weber's *Der Freischütz* immediately springs to mind because of its naked anapest introduction. But this is just one of myriad classical pieces with such a rhythm. Beethoven's symphonies are filled with anapestic rhythms, and the last movement of his glorious Seventh Symphony is practically an homage to the anapest. This is the movement that Wagner couldn't help dancing to. For those who may fear the malefic influence of this deleterious rhythm, I suggest you place your hand over the following figure which is the rhythm that these music healers despise:

Figure 2

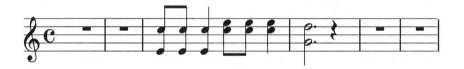

From the Bauern-Marsch of *Der Freischütz* by C. M. von Weber.

Many New Age music healers express fears about the potency of popular music. Halpern's unsupported claim of depressed sexual libido in musicians due to the powerful beat of rock music, and his complaint about the anapestic rhythm, is just one more example of the puritanical fears aroused by the honest expression of the importance of sexual desire and fulfillment in human beings. The Godwins (Jeff and Joscelyn, unrelated and in separate books) express their beliefs that rock 'n' roll is un-Christian.[84] Whether or not this is so, if it has a good beat, teenagers will dance to it. Dance is a worldwide phenomena, in Christian and heathen societies. It is the rare puritanical and repressive culture that forbids dance. Frantic and sexually suggestive dancing is a part of cultures from New York to New Delhi and three thousand or more years of misguided (and mostly unsuccessful) attempts to suppress it should demonstrate—at least to the New Age music healer—that attempts to quash it are more a commentary on the sexual repressiveness of the prohibitionists than a useful method of birth control or moral persuasion.

In his two books, *Dancing with Demons* and *The Devil's Disciples*, Jeff Godwin explicitly states that rock 'n' roll is satanic, that "even the most skeptical person would have to admit . . . that the Devil and rock 'n' roll are good friends." Godwin opines that the "demons [that] John Lennon consorted with . . . possessed Mark David Chapman." The righteous Godwin concludes that, "Lennon had outlived his usefulness as the Devil's slave, and he ceased to exist."[85] It is difficult to read Godwin's comments on Lennon and Lennon's murderer as anything other than a rationalization and approval of a cruel slaying. Even assuming that Godwin has a special knowledge of satanic possession, where is the Christian ethic of "caritas" and compassion?

Laurel Keyes, in *Toning, The Creative Power of the Voice*, chooses to use Lowell Hart's *Satan's Music Exposed* (a book in the same mold as Jeff Godwin's two hysterical polemics) as a source for her anecdotal evidence, which, she believes, shows the evil of rock 'n' roll.

A missionary in Africa experimented with recordings of semi-classical music and acid-rock. He played both to a tribe that had never heard white man's music before. When they listened to semi-classical and harmonic music they responded with smiles and nods of approval and were calm and peaceful. Then, without comment, rock was played. Immediately they reacted. They became agitated. Some grabbed their spears and were ready to fight. Others threw rocks at the record player, apparently trying to kill the threatening thing.[86]

This rather silly anecdote unfortunately depends on racist Western stereotypes of ignorant Africans made popular in Tarzan movies. It is embarrassing that Keyes would credit such a bogus story as that created by Hart (and in 1982) in order to condemn rock 'n' roll. Where in Africa might this have occurred other than the anachronistic Africa of old movies and television? The picture of Africans with spears, throwing rocks at a record player is offered not as comedy but as anecdotal evidence of rock 'n' roll's negative qualities. Keyes is certainly aware that Africans have not "grabbed their spears," then "prepared to fight" since long before Elvis. A glance at the newspaper on almost any given day will show that, unfortunately, when "prepared to fight," Africans are in possession of the same armament that is available to Europeans; and a "tribe" that throws rocks at a record player would most assuredly throw rocks whether the phonograph produced the music of Beethoven or the Beatles. Further debilitating to this anecdotal evidence is the fact that most African traditional music relies heavily on percussion and dance; and rock 'n' roll's roots, most will agree, are planted in the Afro-American musical tradition which in turn derives from the African tradition.

Numerous New Age music healers believe that jazz, blues, rock 'n' roll, and classical music are unhealthy, but none attack them with half the wit and vigor of Joscelyn Godwin. In his book, *Harmonies of Heaven and Earth*, he entertains the reader with thunderous sermons on hellfire and damnation. "The Devil's musical skill serves one purpose only: the seduction of souls. He inverts the purpose of God-given harmony, using the power of music to drag the soul not up but down."[87] Godwin shares Keyes's, Gore's, Halpern's, and Jeff Godwin's righteous indignation with rock music, making clear that rock 'n' roll does not belong to heaven or earth.

> The melodies of plainsong and polyphonic music made the human voice sound like the voice of an angel. Those of opera make it sound like a superman. The Lieder-singer sounds like a lyric poet. And the melodies of popular music? I search the dial of my radio for a random

sampling of current predilections and hear several whores, two her-
maphrodites in distress, a street-fighter, and a few lachrymose labour-
ers. I would not let them into my house: who would want to let such
voices, sinister carriers of psychic influences, into their minds?[88]

And he reports that classical music performances are not devoid of
evil influence either.

At live concerts [clairvoyants] did not just enjoy the visions of beauty
which the music throws off into the air above the stage. . . . They also
saw the concert-hall beset by spirits of ugliness: vile spider-like beings
who swarm around whenever beauty is manifest, and crawl into our ears
and noses while we are entranced by it. . . . During recording, however
it is only the beautiful forms who enter the microphone and whose fair
corpses litter the grooves of our records. The ugly spirits are absent, and
so the full artistic experience is lacking.[89]

It is important to keep in mind when digesting Godwin that he does
not cite the experiences of "clairvoyants" as imagination. Godwin
believes that the "clairvoyants" are simply more accurate reporters of
actual phenomena than those of us who did not notice the arachnoid entities at the symphony. Despite the fact that Godwin informs us that ugly
spirits are not present in the recorded versions of classical music, he
nonetheless advises the reader not to listen to recordings but to attend the
live concert. It is difficult to comprehend this suggestion in light of his
opinion that our ears and noses will be invaded by "spirits of ugliness"
during the time we spend entranced by the music. On the other hand, from
Godwin's descriptions, listening to any music under any conditions seems
risky. If vile, spiderlike beings crawling into our ears and noses is an
essential part of the aesthetic experience, it might be best to spend more
time in our gardens, where real spiders can enter our ears and noses. At
least in our gardens we should be free of the biased, anecdotal claims and

the pseudoscientific speculations of the New Age music healer. But, alas, even there we are not.

Plant Music

One of the most absurd claims of popular pseudoscience is the attribution of mental processes to members of the vegetable kingdom. That they have no apparatus for cognition is overlooked by those who have foisted their unfounded claims on an unsuspecting public. First put forth by the authors Peter Tompkins and Christopher Bird in *The Secret Life of Plants* (which is nothing more than a reworking of a clever Roald Dahl science fiction story titled "The Sound Machine"), the nonsense of consciousness in plants was related as the conclusion of scientifically controlled experiments. Tompkins and Bird have been revealed as frauds whose "experiments" have never been successfully duplicated (though one experimenter did get results using jello instead of plants). For those who have assumed *The Secret Life of Plants* to be a scientifically valid research book I recommend Arthur Galston and Clifford Slayman's article, "Plant Sensitivity and Sensation" in *Science and the Paranormal.*[90]

The Secret Life of Plants attributes "many mental capabilities previously regarded as limited to gods, human beings, and some higher animals" to plants. These include the ability to perceive and respond to human thoughts and emotions, as well as to distant traumatic events, such as the injury or death of other organisms. The book fashions a case for the ability of plants to count, to communicate with each other, and to receive signals from life forms elsewhere in the universe.[91] These unsubstantiated reports were based upon uncontrolled experiments, random observations, and anecdotal reports. The sole "scientific" support for the contentions contained in *The Secret Life of Plants* was the experimental work of polygraph expert Cleve Backster, who followed the "reactions" of plants to various stimulation, including music, with a polygraph machine. Backster jumped to the erroneous conclusion that because the polygraph's output resembled, in a single respect, human records obtained during emotional reaction, the plant must experience something like human emotion. This is roughly equivalent to arguing that because the face of the full moon displays dark patches resembling a human face, there must be a real man in the moon. Polygraph machines will record something no matter what is being tested. Though the "Backster Phenomenon" is nothing more than fiction, Steven Halpern and a number of his followers contend that "sufficient experiments have been performed"[92] to readily accept plants' "emotional" responses to music as scientific fact.

Halpern has latched on to *The Secret Life of Plants* and used it to support his music-healing philosophy and to sell his brand of New Age music. In his second book, *Sound Health*, Halpern reports on research that measured plant polygraph responses to various genres of music. He boasts that the Psychotronics Research Institute, in 1973, found that plants preferred his "Spectrum Suite" to "any other music we were able to test."[93] Interestingly, this Psychotronics Research Institute is the same group that Halpern cites (depending on the book) as concluding in 1973 that Halpern's "Spectrum Suite" was the most relaxing piece of music of all time according to the criteria of the U.S. Surgeon General's office. Both Backster and the Psychotronics group (as described by Halpern) used the same testing equipment, a polygraph. Perhaps they should have asked the plants if they were lying about their musical preference in order to please the researcher.

As the theories on the polygraph responses of plants spin outward from Backster's work they become even more absurd and unrelated to any truth. Dorothy Retallack's *The Sound of Music and Plants* draws heavily upon the dubious research from *The Secret Life of Plants* and is a common source for music-healing philosophy.[94] Both of these books are reported as fact by Joscelyn Godwin. Godwin recognizes that Tompkins, Bird, and Retallack are not really biological experts but excuses their lack of knowledge, calling them "practical," not "theoretical" scientists. Godwin may be ignorant of the fact that "practical" scientists, those that perform physical experiments, have refuted quite definitely in real, "practical" experiments the reported results in *The Secret Life of Plants*. But Godwin dismisses science completely at one point, concluding, "and of course no devoted gardener needs any statistics to prove that plants have feelings."[95] Of course, the most devoted gardener must disregard any feelings plants may have when it comes time to uproot, slice, dice, and eat his green friends.

David Tame is a music healer who cites Retallack's experiments to support his music-healing philosophy in his book, *The Secret Power of Music*. He writes,

> Mrs. Retallack played the music of the two different Denver radio stations to two groups of petunias. The radio stations were KIMN (a rock station) and KLIR (a semi-classical station). The *Denver Post* reported: "The petunias listening to KIMN refused to bloom. Those on KLIR developed six beautiful blooms. By the end of the second week, the KIMN petunias were leaning away from the radio and showing very erratic growth. The petunia blooms hearing KLIR were all leaning toward the sound. Within a month all plants exposed to rock music died."
>
> In another experiment, conducted over three weeks, Dorothy Retallack played the music of Led Zeppelin and Vanilla Fudge to one group of beans, squash (marrow), corn, morning glory and coleus; she also played a contemporary avant-garde atonal music to a second group; and, as a control, played nothing to a third group. Within ten days, the plants exposed to Led Zeppelin and Vanilla Fudge were all leaning away from the speaker. After three weeks they were stunted and dying. The beans exposed to the "new music" leaned 15 degrees from the speaker and were found to have middle-sized roots. The plants left in silence had the longest roots and grew the highest. Further, it was discovered that plants to which placid, devotional music was played not only grew two inches taller than plants left in silence, but also leaned towards the speaker.[96]

Though Retallack's (and Backster's) studies have been shown to be unsubstantiated and bad science, this reality has escaped the attention of music healers. That is a fault in and of itself that infects the music-healing field, but aside from the studies' failures there is a larger issue raised by the music healers' acceptance of Retallack's underlying philosophy that plants are excellent judges of music. For now, I will put aside my objections to the studies themselves and, for the sake of argument, assume that the plant studies were carried out in a valid and scientific manner in order to challenge the issues inherent in the experiments' philosophy.

The plant experiments' results show that petunias thrive when exposed to semiclassical music and die when exposed to rock 'n' roll. Music healers have concluded from this that petunias prefer semiclassical music to rock 'n' roll, and therefore semiclassical music is better than rock 'n' roll. But the fact that one person prefers Wagner to Tchaikovsky does not prove that Wagner is better than Tchaikovsky. Hence, the fact that petunias prefer semiclassical to rock reveals nothing but the petunias' preference, unless one presupposes that petunias are inherently more objective in their response to music than human beings. To date, no New Age music experimenter has tested whether petunias are more objective in their musical preferences than humans.

Bypassing that objection, I will assume (again, for the sake of argument) that it has been proven that petunias are more objective than human beings. Then it needs to be discovered whether what is objectively life-enhancing for petunias is objectively life-enhancing for human beings. If you plant a fertilized human seed beneath a quarter inch of topsoil, maintain it at a temperature of eighty degrees, and water it daily, you will not produce as healthy a human being as you would a petunia whose fertilized seed received the exact same treatment. Music healers would have us believe that what is objectively good for petunias, as determined by experiments, is consequently objectively good for human beings. The opposite may be the case. A modest knowledge of plant and human physiology informs us that petunias require carbon dioxide in order to survive and produce a waste product of oxygen. Human beings require oxygen to survive and produce a waste product of carbon dioxide. The waste product of plants is a life-sustaining element for human beings and vice versa. When looking at the differences between plants and humans in the harsh light of reality, the assumption that what is healthy for plants will be healthy for humans does not hold water. Actually, a likelier application of the results of plant-music experiments to humankind would be the contrary statement: music that is healthy for plants should be avoided by humans.

Various music healers assert that their experiments prove that specific genres of music are beneficial to plant growth and thus beneficial to human beings. For example, they state that a two-foot-tall petunia is better than a one-foot-tall petunia. But that presumes that height is objectively good, that the larger something is the better chance it has to survive. Neither of these claims has any objective meaning, certainly not for the plants, because when people make judgments on what form of plant is the best they invariably choose the plant form that serves man best. The qualities man prefers in plants may have nothing to do with the relative happiness of the plants involved. Are faster-growing, bigger potatoes better for the potatoes, or for human beings? Which petunias are most likely to be plucked and killed for the aesthetic enjoyment of human beings? The scrawny-looking foot-tall petunias with aesthetically displeasing discoloration, or the two-foot-tall petunias that experimenters claim are "better"? And what of the long-lived dwarf bonsai tree and the relatively faster-growing oak? Does the oak benefit because it grows to immense stature and at a greater pace, thereby gaining the lumberman's attention? If, by objectively good, the plant-music experimenter means longer life, then the stunted growth of the bonsai is of greater benefit than the possibly rapid, accelerated growth of the oak subjected to the semiclassical music of Retalack's experiments. Additionally, if oaks and petunias do not share the same musical preferences, then it is unclear which plant is correct.

Some music healers have understood Retallack's conclusions to imply that plants have intelligence as well as consciousness. If plants are intelligent, might they not lie to us or mislead us? After all, we have been killing and eating them for years. When experimenters like Backster, Retallack, and Halpern torture and send telepathically threatening messages to their subjects, whom they claim are capable of intelligence and compassion, should we assume that their testimony is the truth? If plants are compassionate, as the experimenters claim, and altruistic, might they not skew experimental results purposefully in order to misdirect the experimenters? If a petunia knows that the music of Led Zeppelin could produce in it qualities beneficial to man at the expense of the torturous and brief lives of its fellow petunias, might it not prefer a quick and painless suicide to the revelation of its hidden properties valuable to human beings?

And finally, might not the tortured petunias martyr themselves in order to convince humans to listen to music which will ultimately shorten the time human beings hold cruel dominion over the planet, whose living beings they have enslaved and exterminated for the last ten thousand years? Maybe prolonged exposure to New Age music is the key to the plants' "final solution" for the human being problem.

Despite the unsupported, unscientific nature of the plant-music studies, and the absurdity of generalizing their results to human behavior, Halpern and his music-healer colleagues continue to cling to these plant studies, drawing their own various, spurious conclusions. The plant studies offer music healers a proof that human experiments are not likely to provide: that specific genres of music could be defined as objectively bad for humankind, and that a specific genre of music could be objectively good for humankind: the ultimate "healing" music.

In *The Secret Power of Music*, David Tame states clearly the conclusions he has drawn from the plant-music studies.

> Besides the ancients' belief that music affects the body, emotions and mind of man, they also claimed that music's power was *objective*, not subjective. That is, they claimed that different types of music are *inherently good or inherently bad*; that certain combinations of tones are

objectively life-enhancing and evolutionary in nature, while others are unhealthy and dangerous. Should the ancients' belief be true and Mrs. Retallack's work suggests this to be the case, then it would be a fact of vital significance. No longer could modern musicians possibly claim that music is a matter of "taste," or that the musician should be allowed to perform anything he chooses. Moreover, those types of music which are objectively good or objectively bad might not always be found to conform to people's own subjective likes and dislikes. Since all types of music are liked by some individuals and disliked by others, it stands to reason that there must be instances where objectively bad music is nevertheless "liked" by a certain misguided segment of society. Plant-music research, then, in supporting the ancient wisdom teaching on the objective power of music, apparently disproves in one sweep the entire contemporary hedonistic, anarchic viewpoint in the arts. In short, it seems to offer to us a scientific basis from which a permanent and inflexible aesthetics of music can be constructed. Permanent and inflexible because true aesthetic principles are not subjective, but, as we noted in the previous chapter, are universal. Good music is still good music even if there is no human listener.[97]

In the above excerpt, Tame is unabashedly suggesting that the coerced control of people who disagree is a good idea. He asserts that contemporary composers cannot claim that music is a matter of individual preference and insists that musicians should not be allowed to perform the music of their own choice. Tame's music-healing philosophy states that aesthetic principles are objective. People who listen to music that Tame would have us believe is objectively bad are, simply, misguided.

But who does Tame suggest to choose the music of this great new society? Who should determine what musicians are allowed to perform? Tame answers us not with who, but with what: plants. In claiming that music is not an art but rather an objective science Tame denies room for personal freedom of choice. He abdicates our aesthetic choices in favor of those of petunias.

Underlying Tame's desire to install a new social order through the enforcement of compulsory music selection by petunias is a basic and disturbing philosophy that appears to be universally accepted by New Age music healers. It is a philosophy that assumes that human beings should not be permitted the "hedonistic, anarchic" pleasure of listening to music that they enjoy. New Age music healers rally against various genres of music, some attacking rock 'n' roll, some jazz, some classical. Some even attack other music healers' music. Their prohibitions range from the general, as in the Godwins' universal condemnation of rock 'n' roll, to the specific, wherein Diamond says "no" to the Doors, but "yes" to the Beatles. Halpern finds all classical music lacking, whereas Tame gives bravos to Wagner but boos to Mussorgsky. With rare exception the music healer claims the petunia-like ability to evaluate the objective worthiness of music and sound for "appropriate" purposes. Music is thus denied the aesthetic property of subjectivity and becomes an objective science.

Music healers utilize plant experiments to support their criticism of specific genres as "bad" or "unhealthy," and as proof that their own brand of music is "good" or "healthy" or "healing." In a reductio ad absurdam argument, Laurel Keyes sees Retallack's plant experiments as proof that there is an objectively correct music to listen to that is the same not only for petunias as well as people, but also for all matter. She says, "More than any other outside factor, music governs our emotions. . . . This is not through conditioning or imposed attitudes. Experiments made by Dorothy Retallack . . . proved how plants were killed by some music and others flourished with different music. Surely plants do not respond because of "opinions." It was reaction of the molecular structure to the vibrations of sound."[98]

Keyes's reduction finally removes the concept of music from the realm of consciousness altogether. In her philosophy, what we think about what we hear is completely irrelevant to the effect the sound is having upon our molecular structure. This is the ugly truth behind the New Age music healers' philosophy. Theirs is not a philosophy of expanded consciousness, but rather, a narrowing of consciousness to the point where consciousness itself becomes irrelevant. The music healer reduces us to biological robots incapable of aesthetic judgement and the subjective appreciation of art. If we are incapable of selecting music that is good for us, in fact, very likely to pick music that is harmful, then the music healer/composer has the perfect answer: to listen to their music whether we like it or not. Even if we find the music uninspiring, unenlightening, or uninteresting, that's only our brains talking, not our molecules.

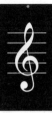

5. Acoustics: Right Understanding

The science of music is acoustics, and no New Age music healer fails to assert that his particular brand of musical nostrum is supported by a firm grasp and application of acoustical principles. Proclaiming expertise belied by their fundamental misunderstanding of the very basic elements of acoustics, they escape detection through the public's understandable lack of knowledge in the field. Doctors, performers, members of the healing professions, music listeners, and even composers have no obligation to understand the science of music in order to appreciate it, to perform it, or to use it for therapeutic purposes. But the same cannot be said for the music healer, who intends to confer acceptability of his pet formulas when he claims that they are acoustically sound. We would not allow our neighbor, no matter how good a person he is, to perform heart surgery upon us, unless he was learned in the field of cardiology. Yet music healers ask us to trust our health to their techniques based upon expertise in a field that their writings and practice show to be nonexistent.

The core of the argument against bogus music-healing techniques is of a technical nature, which, at times, may make it difficult reading for those unfamiliar with acoustics. The focus upon numerical discrepancies is not trivial but serves to prove the fundamental erroneousness of the music healer's healing philosophy. When John Beaulieu informs us that he can cure our ills by playing pitches whose frequencies he has determined by Pythagorean temperament, should we consider him incompetent when we discover that he has incorrectly surmised the frequencies of his healing pitches? Beaulieu tells us that for his healing method to succeed, these frequencies must be tuned to Pythagorean temperament, and yet they are not. Without exception, the music healer does not succeed in meeting his own criteria for healing sounds. Beaulieu's Pythagorean healing forks are not Pythagorean. Kay Gardner's authentic Indian healing ragas are neither authentic nor Indian. Donald Campbell's ameliorative Greek mode improvisations are not in Greek modes. R. J. Stewart's mystical dominant seventh chord is not a dominant seventh chord, and so on. As New Ager Randall McClellan writes, "An understanding of the harmonic series is absolutely essential to the utilization of music as a healing agent."[1] The patient reader will discover that no New Age music healer, including McClellan, can satisfy this rudimentary requirement.

Acoustics

To appreciate Mozart one need not understand the science of acoustics; but to claim acoustical science as the bulwark for a pet theory requires that the theorist truly understand his or her field. Many New Age music healers busy themselves in arcane theorizing based, they say, on the purity of the acoustical foundations of sound; yet they do not properly understand the very acoustics they wish to manipulate for their purposes.

Musical systems of all cultures are based on the physics of sound. If a science fiction author writes about ineffably beautiful music of an extraterrestrial culture based on a completely alien system of acoustics, then he is not familiar with the nature of sound. Underwater, in a concert hall, on the shores of Lake Titicaca, or on a planet with an atmosphere composed of ammonia and methane, the basic principles of acoustics remain the same, though the different environments of the four hypothetical concert settings have significant effects on audition.

Sound travels at 1,087 feet per second in air, but at 4,714 feet per second in water. It travels faster in the same medium depending on temperature (density). At 20 degrees Centigrade sound travels 43 feet per second faster in air than at 0 degrees. The speed of sound, however, has no effect on the frequency of a sound (except in regard to the Doppler effect, but since we are assuming that the listener to New Age music is not required to listen to music as he scurries back and forth from a sound source, we will not explore the ramification of this exception). Frequency is the measurement of pitch as determined by the cycles per second (cps, or hertz: Hz) of a vibrating object. Simply put, if you strike a tuning fork, it wobbles. You can see the wobbling as a blur. You can hear it as sound. The blur is the prong of the tuning fork going back and forth. If it goes back and forth 440 times in one second, its "pitch," by convention, is called "A." (However, A can be quite different. For example, some orchestras prefer tuning to A 435 Hz, some to A 446 Hz; and some to whatever the first oboist considers A that particular performance.) The actual sound is nothing more than the excitation of a medium (in our case: air) by a vibrating object. The tuning fork excites the air surrounding it. This excitation proceeds through the air like a series of falling dominoes until it reaches our ear. Our eardrum is pushed by the excited air just as the air next to the sound source has been pushed, and we hear the sound.

The tuning fork produces a pure tone after it has been struck. (The striking produces a short-lived auxiliary sound, this is not important for our purposes.) Musical instruments, the human voice, and most vibrating systems do not produce pure tones. They produce tones and their harmonics. These harmonics are the basis for tonality and music in every culture because they determine what sounds "good" to the ear. What sounds "good" is no culturally conditioned consensus idea, but a physical reality; but to understand what is "good" one must understand what harmonics are. Since tuning forks are built to suppress harmonics, they cannot serve our purpose any longer. Let us give the tuning fork to the oboist, and turn to the first cellist of the orchestra.

The cello has four strings which, when bowed, plucked, or hit with a stick, vibrate, and thereby cause sound. The thickest string on the cello is the C string. If the cellist has tuned his instrument to A 440 then his C string will vibrate at about 66 Hz. The whole string bounces back and forth 66 times a second, but it also bounces back to a lesser degree in halves, thirds, fourths, fifths, and so on. These lesser divisions of the string create sounds that are called *harmonics*. The 66 Hz C is the fundamental. The lesser sound created by the division of the string in halves is called the second harmonic (there is no "first" harmonic, as the second harmonic is also called the first overtone, but this becomes inordinately confusing, so I will use the terminology of "harmonics"). The sound created by the division in thirds is called the third harmonic, and so on. For the most part, we do not hear the harmonics as distinct pitches, but they contribute to our impression of the timbre of a sound. A cello's C string sounds different than a tuba's C of the same pitch in large part because of the strength of individual harmonics. (There are other factors, principally, the envelope, but I am ignoring these other aspects for the purpose of our discussion of what makes things sound "good.") Certain harmonics will be stronger than others in different types of instruments because of the way they are built, the materials used, and the method of sound production. The clarinet, because it is a closed-tube instrument (as opposed to the flute, which is an open tube instrument) produces a fundamental tone with stronger odd harmonics than even.[2] Though the harmonics are not heard as distinct pitches, harmonics are real and affect our audition of sound. This can be demonstrated easily if a piano is handy. Here is a simple demonstration:

Silently depress and hold the keys middle C, the E a third above, and the G a third above E on a piano. This lifts the hammers from the strings in the piano so that they can vibrate if properly stimulated. Strike briefly and with force the C two octaves below the middle C. You will hear the triad C-E-G after the C has ceased sounding. What has happened is that the fourth, fifth, and sixth harmonics of the C have caused the C, E, and G strings to sympathetically resonate. Notice also how weak the sound is, demonstrating the relative weakness of the harmonics in relation to their fundamental.

Our cellist, sitting patiently, is ready to play. The whole string vibrating freely at 66 Hz produces the C notated:

Figure 3

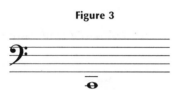

Vibrating in half doubles the hertz to 132, and produces the second harmonic:

Figure 4

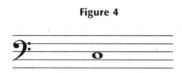

The cellist can produce this tone by placing his finger halfway up the C string and pressing. Thus, cutting the string in half produces a pitch an octave above the open string. If he cuts the string in half yet again the resultant pitch is 264 Hz, the fourth harmonic:

Figure 5

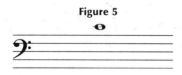

Cleaving the string in half yet again produces the eighth harmonic, vibrating at 528 Hz:

Figure 6

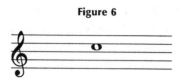

Once more halving produces the sixteenth harmonic, 1,056 Hz:

Figure 7

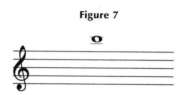

Soon our cellist is running out of room for further doubling, because his finger is not a true geometric point. If his finger was not so clumsy a thing he could continue ad infinitum until Zeno of Elea would scream "Uncle." However, after only five more equal divisions of the string (33,792 Hz), no human being could hear the resultant pitch.

Here then is an incomplete harmonic series:

Figure 8

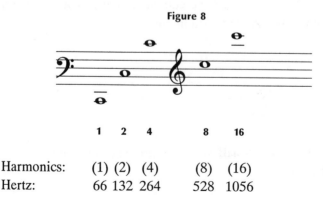

	1	2	4	8	16
Harmonics:	(1)	(2)	(4)	(8)	(16)
Hertz:	66	132	264	528	1056

So far we have only doubled frequency, by cutting in half the string length repeatedly. To complete the harmonic series to the sixteenth harmonic (an arbitrary though not real limit regarding the harmonics above the fundamental pitch) we must divide the string in whole-number ratios. Dividing the string in half doubled the hertz from 66 to 152. Dividing the string in thirds triples the fundamental pitch to 198 Hz. Dividing the string into fifths quintuples the hertz to 330. Here then is the harmonic series, from fundamental through 16th harmonic:

Figure 9

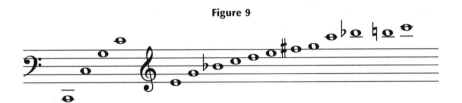

Now we can proceed to discussing what sounds "good." For something to sound "good" one must hypothesize a definition for "good," in music. The best definition is "in agreement." A pitch that is in agreement with another pitch makes a sound that is "good." "Agreement" is compatibility. The pitches, in order to agree, must be compatible. They must be capable of being sounded simultaneously without disturbing each other.

A pitch is not in agreement with another pitch when it is out of tune. Imagine another cellist, arriving late, who has failed to tune up with our oboist, who is on break. This second cellist sits down and joins our first cellist in playing C, but whereas he is playing a C of 66 Hz, she plays a C that vibrates 71 times a second. His 66-Hz tone and her 71-Hz tone played simultaneously cause a phenomena known as "beats." Beats result from the "interference" of two sound waves of slightly different frequencies. There will be five beats per second produced by 66- and 71-Hz sound sources, four beats between 66 and 70 Hz, and so on. The beats are audible as brief amplitude intensifications and are, in the minds of nearly all people of every culture, unpleasant. Even an untrained listener upon hearing two instruments played out of tune, and causing beats, knows that something is wrong. Beats grow in unpleasantness from five or six to about thirty and then decrease in unpleasantness as the beats become too rapid to distinguish. Below five beats per second the sound is not unpleasant. In fact, the "lush" sound of a string section is caused by the beats created as a result of imperfect intonation and is a desired effect.

Our latecomer cellist, recognizing the intonation difficulty, tunes her instrument and now produces a C of 66 Hz. The five-beat-per-second sound is gone. Not only are the fundamentals in agreement, but the harmonics, too. While she played a 71-Hz C and he played a 66-Hz C, the resultant harmonics were out of tune, even more:

	66-Hz C	71-Hz C	Beats
Fundamental	66	71	5
2nd harmonic	132	142	10
3rd harmonic	198	213	15
4th harmonic	264	284	20
5th harmonic	330	355	25
6th harmonic	396	426	30

If we accept "good" as being compatible, then no sounds can be more compatible than the unison, that is, the sounding of one pitch with itself by another sound source. Compatibility will take into consideration harmonic compatibility, making the second-most compatible sound the octave:

Tone #1		Tone #2	
Fundamental	66 Hz		
2nd harmonic	132 Hz	Fundamental	132 Hz
3rd harmonic	198 Hz		
4th harmonic	264 Hz	2nd harmonic	264 Hz
5th harmonic	330 Hz		
6th harmonic	396 Hz	3rd harmonic	396 Hz
7th harmonic	462 Hz		
8th harmonic	528 Hz	4th harmonic	528 Hz
9th harmonic	594 Hz		
10th harmonic	660 Hz	5th harmonic	660 Hz
11th harmonic	726 Hz		
12th harmonic	792 Hz	6th harmonic	792 Hz
13th harmonic	858 Hz		
14th harmonic	924 Hz	7th harmonic	924 Hz
15th harmonic	990 Hz		
16th harmonic	1,056 Hz	8th harmonic	1,056 Hz

The above chart demonstrates that the 66-Hz harmonics are in "agreement" with the 132-Hz harmonics. Octaves are clearly the most agreeable intervals after unisons. Cultures reflect this in their harmonic development. Unison singing is the most primitive harmonic structure. The next level of development is the octave. Following the octave is the first venture into harmonic tension: the third harmonic, a harmonic practice in which a melody is sung with itself a perfect fifth above simultaneously. Harmonic compatibility decreases:

Tone #1		Tone #2	
Fundamental	66 Hz		
2nd harmonic	132 Hz		
3rd harmonic	198 Hz	Fundamental	198 Hz
4th harmonic	264 Hz		
5th harmonic	330 Hz		
6th harmonic	396 Hz	2nd harmonic	396 Hz
7th harmonic	462 Hz		
8th harmonic	528 Hz		
9th harmonic	594 Hz	3rd harmonic	594 Hz
10th harmonic	660 Hz		
11th harmonic	726 Hz		
12th harmonic	792 Hz	4th harmonic	792 Hz
13th harmonic	858 Hz		
14th harmonic	924 Hz		
15th harmonic	990 Hz	5th harmonic	990 Hz
16th harmonic	1,056 Hz		

Following the harmony of the perfect fifth (the third harmonic) is the perfect fourth, which is really only yet another octave above the fundamental. And here the path of music toward greater dissonance becomes rather complex. The fifth harmonic and the sixth harmonic appear in harmonies of some cultures; the seventh (with some acoustical alteration) was essential to the beginnings of Western art music.

Pythagoras and the Harmonic Series

Don Campbell

Don Campbell in *The Roar of Silence* quotes his composition teacher's erroneous concept of progress in harmonic language as measured by the addition of higher harmonics as time has progressed from "antiquity."[3] Nadia Boulanger, Campbell's teacher, believed that harmony is analogous to evolution, not Darwin's valid theory of natural selection, but the anti-Darwinian concept of "higher" and "lower" evolution, a view in which man is placed on the pinnacle of an evolutionary pyramid. This is just species chauvinism, as the mosquito in Darwinian theory is just as "evolved" as man.

In addition, Boulanger and Campbell are confusing harmony with the harmonic series. Harmony and the harmonic series are not identical. In Boulanger's contrived scheme, Western man is most evolved because his harmonic language includes simultaneous intervals which are found higher in the harmonic series than most other harmonic languages of the world. Generations of music theory teachers have witnessed classes founder on this very confusion between harmony and harmonics in the evolution of music in various cultures worldwide.

Every tribe, every community, every culture on earth has music. There are many different varieties of music and there are many ways that each tribe, community, and culture produces a musical language. Painful as it may be to New Age music theoreticians, there is no tuning system, no musical language in the world based solely upon the natural harmonic series. The harmonic series itself is not a scale as Boulanger and Campbell assume. If the harmonic series were a scale, wouldn't it be called the harmonic scale? Every musical language uses an artificial, *man-made* scale in order to determine which pitches are to be used within an octave. This is not as silly as it sounds. There are infinite choices of pitches within an octave. The pitches chosen by each culture in devising their musical language is that culture's "temperament" system. Campbell and Boulanger's theory that our Western equal temperament system is more evolved than other cultures is shown to be fallacious and chauvinist in light of the reality that many non-Western cultures (such as India) use higher harmonics in their construction of musical systems than does the Western musical system. Western equal temperament is no more evolved than the tuning systems of Ghana, Thailand, Java, or India. It is Campbell's and Boulanger's prejudice in regard non-Western cultures that causes them to assume that the tuning systems of other cultures are less sophisticated than our own Western tuning systems.

There is no correlation in a culture's use of harmony and its application of the harmonic series to its temperaments. The folk music of a culture most clearly demonstrates this truism.

Several Eastern European and Pacific tribes use dissonant "advanced" sonorities (simultaneous intervals of less than a major second), yet construct their basic scales using tunings based on intervals obtainable from the first twelve harmonics. Contrarily, much folk music of Western Europe which is chromatic (and equal tempered) never uses simultaneous sonorities of less than a major second, except as non-harmonic passing tones or appogiaturas. (For examples, see Sachs's *Wellsprings of Music*.[4] His examples from Lithuanian and Polynesian polyphony are quite striking.) What Boulanger and Campbell have done is to confuse harmony with the harmonic series and then confer specious qualities of technological progress on this concept.

R. J. Stewart

In *Music and the Elemental Psyche* R. J. Stewart shows that he is unaware that "artificial" tunings are a part of numerous cultures for numerous reasons and are not restricted to Western classical music. He writes, "The modern alterations of temper or relativity [*sic*] between notes are mainly due to certain mechanistic problems in the development of keyboard instruments."[5] Not only is this assertion evidence of ignorance of folk musics of the world, it also ignores the Pythagorean tuning he cites frequently as natural, which in fact is as artificial as the tempered system, and which was developed two millennia before the invention of keyboard instruments.

Pythagorean, mean-tone, equal temperament (and the unused, theoretical just intonation) are all artificial systems devised, by man, to accommodate unnatural alterations to the harmonic series. In equal temperament, except for the octave, no interval is natural. The moment one puts a fret on a string or a hole in a tube or gathers a group of people together to sing in different octaves, choices of temperament must be made. When man blew through a tube he could only play notes of the harmonic series; so he cut holes in the tube, put flaps over the holes, and cursed nature with beautiful artifice.

Those holes cut in the tubes presented a problem for man and nature, videlicit: where to put the holes. Curt Sachs explains in *The Wellsprings of Music*:

> The holes appear in strange arrays. It is obvious—as every violinist or guitarist knows—that two musical steps of equal width require different strides on the instrument, with the second smaller than the first one, and so forth. This applies to finger holes as much as to frets: their progression should be, in mathematical language, "harmonic" rather than "arithmetic." But no array of holes proceeds in a harmonic progression; the holes are equidistant throughout or else arranged in two groups, either one with equidistant holes and separated from one another by a somewhat larger space. And often the holes begin only in the exact middle of the flute and leave the upper half intact. . . . It is, to be true, not only the visual but also the tactile sense to which the ear must yield.[6]

What Stewart and his ilk fail to realize is that due to physiological restraints of the human organism, no intonation system can be natural. In order to fill an octave with pitches, human beings must choose what pitches they want, and how many. Many cultures have chosen five, many seven, and many twelve; as well as six and twenty-two. Not all cultures employ equal-tempered tuning and the music healer who disdains our culture's use of equal temperament will often point to the temperament systems of cultures they perceive as more primitive, hence more natural, as being better for healing. But their lack of knowledge in regard to acoustics is a fatal flaw in their reasoning, because the temperament systems of nearly all the cultures they name are also equal-tempered, only their temperaments are based upon equal-tempered scales of seven or five steps rather than the Western twelve.

Peter Michael Hamel

The fact that Western culture has twelve steps in the octave actually permits the Western composer greater access to the use of intervals closer to the natural harmonic series than those with fewer pitches. India, with its complex, twenty-two *sruti* system, is one of the few practiced temperaments with greater flexibility than the Western twelve-tone system.

A frequent example cited by music healers of a natural tuning system is that used by the Balinese. Yet in actuality, the Balinese tune their five-step scale to equal-tempered steps of 240 cents ("cents" are a logarithmic presentation of interval in which an octave is 1200 cents). "Two south African peoples, Bapendi and Chopi, give their xylophones an iso-heptatonic arrangement with seven equal steps of about 171 cents in an octave, which amounts exactly to the current genders of Siam (Thailand) and Burma," explains Sachs.[7] Regardless of the perceived primitivism of a culture, the vast majority of peoples prefer and construct systems of temperament based upon equal steps. The natural harmonic series, in which each successive step is unique, has proven impractical to every single culture. There is *no* musical practice on the earth in which nature's harmonic series remains pure. Different cultures retain different intervals of the harmonic series and begin to think of these intervals as "natural." But no one harmonic above a fundamental can be said to be any more natural than another. It would be haughty and irrelevant to gloat over the fact that traditional Ugandan folk music does not have as "natural" a perfect fourth and fifth, as does Western culture.

Perhaps music healers are confused because of the "natural" way musicians from other countries tune their instruments. But this "natural" tuning is no more natural than the Western violinist's ability to tune his own instrument. Neither the European violinist nor the Ugandan harpist needs an oscilloscope to tune his instrument to what he perceives as correct. Ugandan harpists tune adjacent strings 240 cents apart by ear using a relatively unnatural perfect fourth of 480 cents. Compare that to the American violinist, who can tune utilizing perfect fourths of 500 cents. The "natural" unaltered perfect fourth is 498 cents. Note that neither the Ugandan harpists nor the Western violinists, in their tuning, are creating a tuning that is "natural."

Peter Hamel, in *Through Music to the Self*, attempts to explain the Indonesian gamelan as foreign to our Western ears because "all the metallophonic and gong-type instruments . . . are alike exactly tuned to . . . unnatural intervals."[8] Indeed, they are unnatural, but so is our Western twelve-note-to-the-octave tuning. Hamel denigrates the individuality of gamelan orchestras. He writes, "The Balinesians have not been overcareful to stick to received tradition, and have written their own 'operas,' " pejoratively describing the rich diversity of gamelan. Hamel believes that Westerners "accustomed as they are to tempered keyboards and harmonics" cannot appreciate the varied musics of the world.[9] Westerners with no exposure to gamelan might find the gamelan "out of tune" or alien, but so would the analogous Indonesian find the classical symphony orchestra and the differently tuned Indian music as well. There is a short-sightedness in Hamel's praise of the foreign, and an implication that the gamelan is better because of its mysteriousness to him, yet he fails to turn the coin over, to examine what he myopically views as "music that has arisen from levels of consciousness other than our own mental one."[10] Western music, he implies is "mental" (whatever that means), but non-European music is—different. Well, yes, of course it is different, but Hamel has fallen into the same chauvinist trap of the European bigot who, seeing non-European culture as different, labeled it inferior. In interesting contrast to Hamel's assertion that Western music is "mental" is William David's equally unwarranted statement that "sounds in the Oriental schools are very precise and mental, with little feeling or emotion."[11]

Curt Sachs relates an edifying story in *The Wellsprings of Music.* In Belgrade, Yury Arbatsky "had taken an excellent Albanian folk musician to Beethoven's Ninth Symphony. Asked how he had liked it, the man hesitated and at last, after a couple of brandies, gave the astonishing answer: 'Fine—but very, very plain (lepo ali preprosto).' The Albanian was neither arrogant nor incompetent. He just has a different standard."[12] Sachs also tells of a "highly educated Chinese lady" who, after being introduced to Mozart's *Requiem,* considered it "superficial"![13] Should we condemn the Albanian or the Chinese? Of course not. Condemning Westerners for a lack of appreciation for ethnic musics, one would expect Peter Hamel to himself show respect for ancient foreign musical tradition, yet in *Through Music to the Self* he does a disservice to the non-Western intonation of Indian ragas by claiming, astonishingly, that they "correspond to the old church modes."[14] He proceeds to list several of them, with pitches of the Western equal-temperament system (which uses twelve pitches per octave as opposed to the twenty-two pitches or *sruti* of Indian music), as well as indicate a completely fictitious method for constructing the rest. What Hamel may have had in mind, though I cannot be sure, is a comparison of some Indian ragas in B. Chaitunya Deva's *Music of India: A Scientific Study,* in which Deva compares thirteen Indian scales to various Western scales and modes; but Deva is comparing them, not equating them; and these thirteen Indian scales are but a small percentage of the five-hundred-odd scales in the Indian repertoire. In addition, of these seven-note scales only two pitches from each Indian scale are actually equatable with the Western scales. However, a superficial reading of Deva's study might leave the acoustical layperson with the impression that Deva is showing the similarities between the scales, when in fact, he was pointing out the great differences between them.

Like many other New Age music theorists Hamel misunderstands the harmonic series. Speaking of the seventh harmonic he notes that it "is regarded by harmonicists as eccentric, or only marginal."[15] First, what is a "harmonicist"? Is it someone who plays the harmonica? Second, the seventh harmonic is no more marginal than the ninth. The seventh harmonic is a prominent element in differentiating the timbres of different instruments. Western equal temperament calls for an intonation in which the seventh partial is radically altered, not "eccentric." Using the useless and deceptive neologism "natural tone-row" instead of the clear and accepted term "harmonic series," Hamel erroneously proclaims, "Normally, however, only the first eleven are used in harmonic research."[16] This is patently false. To believe that only the first eleven harmonics are used in "research" requires us to accept as fact that acoustic researchers never study the instruments of the orchestra. To give an example, French horn players regularly play high pitches by overblowing. To play Mozart's Second Horn Concerto, horn players of the time had to utilize the twelfth through sixteenth partials, as well as the second through eleventh. Some of Hamel's improbable conclusions seem to stem from a lack of understanding of the frequencies and harmonics he enumerates. He creates a table to show how humans speak in different registers, depending on the vowel sound. The sound "oo" he cites as 300 Hz, the sound "ee" as 3000 Hz, with six intermediate ascending frequencies so that it is clear that the difference in range he gives of over three octaves is no typographical error. This range is virtually impossible.

Hamel though, has little time to putter about in the mundane reality of frequencies and intervals, and one might consider his objection to a disregard for the facts as trivial compared to the theosophic tidbits he wishes to impart. "In the the light of scientific research into ultrasound and the properties of ultrasonic tones even the legendary tradition that the Egyptian pyramids were built with the aid of 'chanted spells and deep tones' seems a little less far-fetched than before."[17] For Hamel, the harmonic series is a gateway to a fabulous past in which Pythagoras occupies the role of shaman and priest, not scientist.

Randall McClellan

Most New Age books in which their authors strive to explain the meaning and effect of music begin with the presentation and explication of the harmonic series. This is a logical starting point for any exposition on music. *The Healing Forces of Music*, a "history, theory, and practice" of healing music, by Randall McClellan is no exception. However, McClellan's opening chapter, "The Physical Manifestation of Sound" is seriously flawed. The diagram of the harmonic series is incorrect.[18] The eleventh harmonic is not the right pitch, and the seventh is placed in parentheses for no reason. If McClellan intends to show that the seventh is "out of tune" by most artificial temperament systems then he ought to parenthesize other "out of tune" pitches, notably the eleventh, thirteenth, and fourteenth (the fourteenth is identically out of tune as the seventh, being its octave). This he does not. For no discernable reason he divides the series into six specious segments, with unexplained, gratuitous brackets. At first glance these errors might be attributed to the oversight of a typesetter, if not for further evidence of a general confusion regarding the science of acoustics. McClellan states that harmonics proceed from the fundamental "up to" the sixteenth harmonic. He also states, incorrectly, that "Pythagoras determined that a string vibrates not only as a whole but also in segments of halves, thirds, fourths, fifths, sixths, sevenths, eighths, and so on up to sixteenths."[19] There is that "up to the sixteenth" again. Apparently McClellan believes that a brick wall of silence occurs after the sixteenth harmonic. Teachers of acoustics as a matter of convenience, when demonstrating the principle of the harmonic series, typically stop at sixteen, but not without explaining the potentially infinite progression.

McClellan's insistence that the harmonic series comes to a full stop at the sixteenth harmonic is more than misleading, it betrays a lack of appreciation for the influence of higher harmonics on timbre. In addition, McClellan implies that Pythagoras shared this misunderstanding of the harmonic series by falsely attributing to Pythagoras the quote "up to the sixteenth." These exceptions to McClellan's treatise may seem nothing but nitpicking, but so far we have not even turned past page 15, on which McClellan notes, "The principle [*sic*] tone plus its 'harmonics' results in a sound of incredible richness." Principle or principal (whichever he intends) is a superfluous coinage. The word should be fundamental, but the principal error here is in the assertion that the "incredible richness" is a result of harmonics. *All* fundamentals, with rare exception (such as electronically produced sine tones) have harmonics. Therefore, attributing richness in sound to the presence of harmonics is merely stating that all sounds (with the exception of the electronically produced sine tones) are rich. Is this what he means, simply that all sounds are rich? We must assume not. What McClellan should say is that the relative strength of various harmonics give individual instruments their own particular timbre. Perhaps McClellan thinks a horn sound is "rich," whereas a xylophone sound is not. The difference in the horn and xylophone sound is, in large part, attributable to the relative strengths of the harmonics above the pitches played by these instruments (and several other factors, as well). As both the xylophone and horn produce harmonics, attributing richness to one and not the other because of the presence of harmonics is simply erroneous.

Still, on page 15, McClellan defines "nodes" as the "juncture of the two halves" in a string where "no movement takes place." This is true only for the node of the second harmonic, not for the node of the third, fourth, fifth, or any other harmonic up to, and exceeding, the sixteenth.

On page 16 McClellan returns to the subject of Pythagorean temperament. "It was through the harmonic series that Pythagoras was able to calculate the intervals which were used throughout the Western world until a different, more artificial tuning system was adopted—namely the predecessor of our present equal temperament scale."[20]

First, it was not through the harmonic series that Pythagoras was able to calculate intervals "used throughout the Western world." Pythagoras identified the harmonic series through his experimentation, but he was unfortunately unable to calculate even the intervals used in Greece at the time of his experimentation. The intervals of the Greek modes were not simply a reconstruction of the harmonic series, and the limitations of the technology of Pythagoras's time prevented him from defining the intervalic content of the modes; this was a great loss to history because no one

else could either. The contemporary explanations of the musical temperaments of Pythagoras's period are all merely poetic musings. There is no
Rosetta Stone for revealing the tuning of the Greek modes and thus, we
will never know what the music of Pythagoras's time sounded like.

In fact, there was no uniform set of intervals used throughout the
Western world during Pythagoras's time. There was not even a uniform
set of intervals for the Greek modes themselves, as we know from the
admissions of contemporary poets and musicians who bemoaned the fact
that the tunings for a particular mode in one state were completely different from those in a neighboring state. As for the rest of Europe, they did
not even use the Greek modes.

The temperament that Pythagoras devised was an artificial tuning
based upon the ratio between the frequencies of the second and third harmonics. It is not a natural tuning. In fact, it was an attempt to create a
standard, artificial system that could be easily and logically disseminated
in order to eliminate the confusing and variable tunings of the modes used
during Pythagoras's time. McClellan's confusion is perhaps based on his
mistaken belief that Pythagoras constructed his scale from the intervals
derived from the natural harmonic series, rather than from one single
interval, the perfect fifth, the ratio of 3:2, which is but one of many disparate intervals obtainable from the harmonic series.

And finally, what does McClellan mean by "namely the predecessor
of our present equal temperament scale?" He never names it. What predecessor is he talking about? Why does he call it "more artificial"?
Pythagoras's temperament is artificial; though different than mean-tone
or equal temperament, it is still artificial.

In addition to this errant report on Pythagoras's theory McClellan
includes a chart and mathematical formula for determining the pitch
ratios and frequencies from "Pythagoras's calculations." He says
Pythagoras' octave is a 2:1 ratio. This is correct. So is the ratio of 3:2 for
the fifth. But then McClellan pursues the natural harmonic series ratios
while Pythagoras's actual tunings diverge. McClellan claims that the

Pythagorean major third is a 5:4 ratio. Pythagoras's major third is in actuality 81:64. McClellan claims that the Pythagorean minor second is 16:15. Pythagoras's minor second is 256:243. McClellan's claim for Pythagoras minor third is also wrong, but the point is made.

Finally McClellan offers a formula for figuring out all the intervals of the Pythagorean system that is horribly wrong. It has nothing to do with Pythagoras's formula. For those who note that McClellan's 5:4 ratio is "close" to 81:64 and that 16:15 is "close" to 256:243, understand that Pythagorean temperament is *defined* by these differences. If it seems that the ratio of 81:64 is less "natural" than 5:4, then you have grasped Pythagoras's point. Those who romanticize Pythagoras as some sort of primitivist icon of natural thinking are inventing a person who is the diametric opposite of Pythagoras the man, and what his work represented. The simple ratios that McClellan cites are possible only in an untempered scale. McClellan nullifies the changes Pythagoras deliberately made to the natural harmonic series. In effect, McClellan has invented a Pythagoras who did absolutely nothing, an anti-Pythagoras.

Having reached page 16 there is a temptation to mirror McClellan's own "up to the sixteenth" caveat and turn a deaf ear to further musings; but McClellan has promised more, specifically: "the equal temperament scale." But alas, nowhere in McClellan's book does he fulfill the promise of page 16; nowhere does he name the "predecessor of our present equal temperament scale" or even discuss the presumed successor; but perhaps it is perfectly fitting that he end his attempt at explaining the harmonic series on page 16 and fitting that his reader end here too, for though strange and wondrous worlds await the reader of McClellan's book it is questionable whether any reader is capable of truly understanding McClellan's real message.

Contemplate this: "An understanding of the harmonic series is absolutely essential to the utilization of music as a healing agent."[21] This self-denying quote is McClellan's own footnote to his misrepresentation of the harmonic series, Pythagoras, and other acoustical matters on page 15. I am dumbfounded. The man is merciless in his own condemnation. I would even plead his own case. He need not disqualify himself as a potential healer just because he misunderstands the harmonic series and Pythagoras. After all, he is not the only New Age music healer with this liability.

Dane Rudhyar

Dane Rudhyar confuses the Greek system of modes, which were, according to contemporary writers, a set of tetrachords using different beginning pitches, with a fanciful notion of separate tribal influences.

> It seems evident to me that the earliest modes probably were more than a combination of four or five descending tetrachords with set intervals. They were the complex ways in which particular tribes intoned their sacromagical chants accompanied by simple instruments. . . . The Dorians may have been the main and the last group that invaded Greece proper from northern mountainous valleys, but they undoubtedly mixed with earlier inhabitants, perhaps colonies from the previous Cretan culture. Later, the Dorians themselves colonized the islands of the Aegean Sea (for example, Samos where Pythagoras was born) and the coastal regions of Asia Minor and Southern Italy.[22]

Does Rudhyar not find it curious and extremely unlikely that disparate tribal groups would bring separate modes, invented independently, into one place and that they just happened to fit together into a cohesive, precise, artificial musical style? This thinking is the equivalent of breaking a Grecian urn into eight random fragments, tossing them into the air and assuming that they will fall down together to form the original urn. It could happen, but Rudhyar's theory depends upon just that happening. If Rudhyar were given these eight fragments, would he assume that eight separate tribes made these eight separate shards and then, coincidentally, met in Athens one year and put them together to create the art of the Grecian urn? His assumptions about the Greek modes are precisely this.

In fact, Rudhyar provides a warning regarding this. In *The Magic of Tone and the Art of Music* he writes that "the origins of Christian music are but superficially known."[23] He warns that the Eurocentric view of history has prevented an intelligent inquiry into the music of Asia. This is a wise admonition, but in the same book Rudhyar analyzes ancient and oriental music from the viewpoint of a Westerner ignorant of the fact that ancient Egyptians and Indians did not read Helmholtz nor have complex oscilloscopes available in order to tune their scales. Rudhyar suggests that the ancient Egyptian and Indian eleven notes to the octave scale were derived from "the section of the harmonic series between the eleventh and the twenty-second harmonic."[24] This suggests that the ancient Egyptians and Indians had instruments capable of playing the eleventh through twenty-second harmonics over a fundamental, or had oscilloscopes. It also assumes that these people had a reason for tuning to the eleventh harmonic. Even today's enormous double bass of Western music can barely sound clearly the eleventh, thirteenth, fourteenth, or fifteenth harmonics as natural harmonics. What sort of enormous and facile instruments did Rudhyar assume these ancient peoples had? True, French hornists can sound the sixteenth harmonic, but such an effort is extremely difficult and they do not tune their eleventh harmonic, nor have they ever. Does Rudhyar think the ancient Indians had brass players screeching away at stratospheric pitches merely to tune their instruments? This shows that Rudhyar is unfamiliar with how musical intonation systems develop, the technical restraints of musical instruments, and the physical limitations of the humans who play them.

The simplest intonation system and one of the most prevalent is based upon a 3:2 ratio (the perfect fifth) enunciated by Pythagoras. A stringed instrument, such as the lyre, can be tuned by selecting a starting string and finding the node one third of the way from its end. This enables the string player to hear a pitch an octave and a fifth above the fundamental of the string, and to thus match the pitch of another string whose fundamental is a perfect fifth removed from the first pitch. This procedure can be repeated six times in order to create a seven-pitch scale. A twelve-pitch scale can be derived through five more repetitions, but the resulting octaves will no longer be in tune. Thus, Pythagorean intonation failed to provide a coherent and feasible temperament for Western music once Western music developed a penchant for modulation and chromatic alteration.

But rather than understand his system, Rudhyar paints a picture of a mysterious Pythagoras whose disciples "believe" rather than understand his contributions to music. Pythagoras's system of intonation is not an esoteric or spiritual belief system; it is a simple, mechanistic technique for tuning a scale. What Rudhyar and other music healers see as mystery is not mystery, but only their own less-than-rudimentary knowledge of methods of intonation. Part of this confusion lies in the inability to put aside twentieth-century, Western, equal-temperament pitch classifications while pondering ancient music.

But ultimately Rudhyar reports that "the harmonic series is a myth,"[25] which may explain his misunderstanding of it. On page 56 of *The Magic of Tone and the Art of Music*, Rudhyar shows his version of the harmonic series and labels the intervals incorrectly. He does not differentiate between major thirds and minor thirds nor major seconds and minor seconds. To say that 5:4 defines the "third" is a significant mistake if one does not identify 6:5 as the minor third (and 5:4 as the major third). One cannot use the Western term "third" without differentiating. It is not necessary to relate the harmonic series to Western terms, but if one does use Western terms, one is obligated to use them correctly, or accept that the resulting explanations are reduced to gibberish.

John Beaulieu

Pythagoras seems to weave a spell of enchantment on New Age music theoreticians and composers alike, but it is a spell that precludes real understanding of Pythagoras. John Beaulieu is a music healer whose healing system reveals his misunderstanding of Pythagorean intonation,

Pythagoras, and acoustics. Beaulieu has constructed a theory of "healing and meditating with tuning forks" based on Pythagorean intervals. He writes, "The use of tuning forks in healing and meditation involves three components: extension, intention, and reception. Extension is the *method* [Beaulieu's emphasis] of producing sound. Extension involves understanding the tuning fork system. The forks *must* [my emphasis] be tuned to Pythagorean intervals as follows. . . ." Beaulieu lists them as C = 256 cps, D = 288 cps, E = 320 cps; F = 341.3 cps, G = 384 cps, A = 426.7 cps, B = 439.9 cps, and C = 512 cps.[26]

The problem with Beaulieu's tunings are that they are not Pythagorean. Like many other New Age music healers Beaulieu chose 256 cps as the frequency for C. This is not a frequency for C used by any orchestras or performing groups, but rather a theoretical C designed to help students who are beginning to learn acoustics. The argument, however, is not with Beaulieu's selection of 256 cps, but rather with his inability to apply the Pythagorean technique in the formulation of the other frequencies he lists. To find the Pythagorean frequency for G one should multiply 256 by $\frac{3}{2}$. Beaulieu does this successfully. The next pitch, D, is found by multiplying the frequency of G by $\frac{3}{2}$ and then dividing by $\frac{1}{2}$ yet again to place it in the same octave as the C and the G. This is a slightly more complicated procedure, but one that Beaulieu succeeds, again, in accomplishing. However, at this point Beaulieu no longer remembers this simple formula for extracting pitches in Pythagorean temperament. The pitch A, proceeding as one should, is 432 cps in Pythagorean intonation. But Beaulieu lists 426.7 as the Pythagorean A. The next pitch, E, should be 324 cps calculating from the correct A of 432 cps, but Beaulieu's previous error spawns an incorrect E. B, as calculated from a C of 256 cps should be 486 cps. Even calculating from his previous incorrect E, the figure should be 480 cps, but Beaulieu gives 439.9 cps, which is so far removed from the Pythagorean B, or any B, that I am at a loss to explain this calculation. In fact, 439.9 cps is too low a frequency even for B♭. But Beaulieu compounds his error here by stating that B in Pythagorean temperament should have a frequency

11/12ths that of the C immediately above it. The C immediately above it is 512 cps, therefore the B that does have a frequency 11/12ths of that C would be 469.3 cps, not 439.9 cps. In either case, Beaulieu is wrong when he states that the B in Pythagorean intonation should be 11/12ths the C above it. What Beaulieu is doing here is forgetting that the intervalic relationships between pitches is logarithmic, not arithmetic, so that though B is the eleventh chromatic pitch in the Western scale and C is the twelfth, the intervalic ratio between the two is not 11/12ths. The correct Pythagorean ratio is 243/256. In the harmonic series the B to C ratio is 15/16. Beaulieu is totally at sea regarding Pythagorean intonation.

Beaulieu sells his pretend Pythagorean tuning forks through his "Sound School," but as his entire system of healing is based on a fundamentally flawed interpretation of Pythagorean temperament this flaw raises serious questions about all of his claims. Beaulieu writes, "Extension involves understanding the tuning fork system."[27] His failure to understand Pythagorean intonation and to detect the huge discrepancies between the specific frequencies he claims as necessary for healing and the actual frequencies he uses proves Beaulieu's scheme meritless.

Manly Hall and Steven Halpern

"Long before anything was known of pitch numbers, or the means of counting them," writes Helmholtz in *On the Sensations of Tone*,

> Pythagoras had discovered that if a string be divided into two parts by a bridge, in such a way as to give two consonant musical tones when struck, the lengths of these parts must be in the ratio of these whole numbers. If the bridge is so placed that $\frac{2}{3}$ of the string lie to the right, and $\frac{1}{3}$ on the left, so that the two lengths are in the ration of 2:1, they produce the interval of an Octave, the greater length giving the deeper tone. Placing the bridge so that $\frac{3}{5}$ of the string lie on the right and $\frac{2}{5}$ on the left, the ratio of the two lengths is 3:2, and the interval is a Fifth.[28]

Helmholtz wrote his great book in the nineteenth century. The science of acoustics has advanced, as would be expected, since then, but little of Helmholtz's work is obsolete. Science does march on, however, and in the case of Pythagoras, though much of his work on harmonics is still valid, his theories on the harmony of the heavenly objects are now seen as only wishful thinking. Manly Hall, in his *Philosophy of Music,* is exercising a little wishful thinking of his own when he writes, "Modern musicologists tell us that the mathematical intervals represented by the orbits of the planets, as we know these intervals astronomically, in no way conflict with the Pythagorean concept of the monochordum mind."[29] Thus in one sentence Hall aligns musicology, mathematics, astronomy, Pythagoras, and acoustics to support a claim that is pure fantasy. To illustrate his contention, misleadingly labeled as fact, that Pythagoras's musings are still scientifically accurate, Hall includes an illustration of the "orbits of the planets" with their respective Pythagorean acoustical attributes. Naturally, the earth is shown as the center of this outdated map of the solar system, and the planets and other celestial objects are in inaccurate orbits in relation to each other. Is it asking too much of Hall for him to appreciate that as Pythagoras's calculations for the harmony of the spheres was based upon the false belief that the earth was the center of the solar system it is extremely likely that twentieth-century scientists, be they acousticians or astronomers, would find a conflict between the Pythagorean geocentric harmony of the spheres and the solar system as we know it today?

Steven Halpern bemoans the fact that Pythagoras is known only for having "invented [*sic*] a certain kind of triangle,"[30] and that his music of the spheres is never mentioned. Apparently, a lot of people somehow find out about the music of the spheres. Halpern credits Pythagoras as being "the first to come out of the closet so to speak in recognizing the connection between the seven planets, the seven Greek modes and the seven whole steps in the diatonic scale."[31] The first part of this statement is simply ahistorical. Pythagoras could not have "connected" seven planets with anything because Greek civilization during and for many years after Pythagoras did not know of seven planets. Halpern is just making this up. As for Halpern's "seven whole steps in the diatonic scale," this is just not so. There are five whole steps and two half steps in the diatonic scale, (a total distance of six whole steps in the octave, if one were to count that way.) In regard the seven Greek modes, I assume Halpern is referring to the Dorian mode and its six relatives, a musical system created after Pythagoras's death. Pythagoras could not have known of these seven scales, as the music of his time was based upon tetrachordal systems of four pitches each.

Though Halpern tends to avoid acoustics, he does manage to become entangled in it occasionally. "If the string was plucked at one quarter of its length . . . the string has a point in the middle at which the string is at rest and two more points at which it is attached to the frame. These points are called nodes,"[32] he notes in *Tuning the Human Instrument*. First, what he means to say is that if one places a finger one quarter of the way up a string and then the player plucks or bows the string, there will be created several nodes, or resting places, where the string does not vibrate. These nodes will be at the ends of the string, at the point where the finger touches, and at two other locations (at half and at three-quarters of the length of the string) not simply at the ends and in the middle. The resultant sound will be the fourth harmonic of the fundamental. However, if one follows Halpern's directions and plucks the string one quarter of the way from the end, there will be no nodes on the string (there will be but two nodes at the ends of the string); you will not get the fourth harmonic, nor any other harmonic, there will not be a node at the midpoint of the string, and you will have demonstrated nothing but the effect called pizzicato.

R. J. Stewart

In *Music and the Elemental Psyche*, R. J. Stewart imports Gareth Knight to address the issue of Pythagoras and the harmonic series in "Three Systems of Metaphysical Music," the fifth appendix of his book. He quotes from Knight's *The Rose Cross and the Goddess*:

In the rituals of a certain Order, the Magus of the Lodge states that each of the Officers represents "a note in the chord of the ritual," and the Magus, by contacting each officer, then proceeds "to set that chord vibrating."

That chord we may derive from the harmonics of a vibrating string. . . . This was the device used by the Pythagorean philosophers to explain their philosophical number system.

. . . Dividing a string by 2, we get the so-called octave, or the same note at a higher mode of manifestation. In tonic solfa this will be high *doh*. . . . If we divide the string into 5 we get another important note. This is generally called the "third," or, the tonic solfa system, *me* [*sic*]. An important quality of this note is that it can manifest in one of two ways, each of which gives a different quality of feeling. In conventional musical terms this is called the major or minor mode. And, in very simplified terms, a piece of music will sound bright or sad according to whether the third note of the conventional scale is in the major or minor mode. (In the minor mode the 3rd is flattened.)

In symbolic terms of Pythagorean mathematics and musicology this dual mode of expression introduces the principle of polarity at a new level of expression. It is analogous to sexual or other expressions of polarity in manifestation.

Division by 6 need not detain us here.[33]

Here Gareth Knight succeeds in mystifying some readers, but the highfalutin language is basically a cover-up of his lack of comprehension of Pythagoras and acoustics. When Knight says that the "division of the string into six should not detain us" he is implying a comprehension of the material that his analysis belies. Knight explains that the division of the string into five parts produces the intervals of both the major and the minor third, and claims this as a basis for a magical system of polarity. Knight compromises his magical system by failing to proceed to the division of the string into six which, in fact, provides us with the minor third he inaccurately assigns to the division of the string into fifths. Knight may honestly be confused about the derivation of major and minor thirds, and rightly assume that most of his readers will know less about acoustics than he does. But by fabricating an expertise in acoustics he harms his sponsor, R. J. Stewart, by saddling his book with a pretend chapter on acoustics. Knight could have assisted Stewart by taking the time to research the relevance of the fourth, fifth, and *sixth* partials to the derivation of the major and minor third.

Barbara Anne Scarantino

"Music, the very word is music to my ears," begins Barbara Anne Scarantino's *Music Power, Creative Living through the Joys of Music*. Like McClellan's work, the opening pages of Scarantino's book contain some "Pythagorean" theory.

> The combinations of sounds that we hear and call "music" are also created by applying certain rules of mathematics set forth by Pythagoras who, as you will recall, studied all the rhythms and cycles of the universe and created the formula for music as we know it.
>
> These mathematical principles are evident in every aspect of music (scales, chords, time signatures, tempos, and rhythms) and have a corresponding "cosmic connection." For example, Pythagoras developed the seven tones of the scale (do-re-me-fa-so-la-ti) by calculating the distance from the moon to the earth (one tone), the distance from the moon to Mercury (semitone), from Mercury to Venus (one and a half tones), the sun to Mars (one tone), Mars to Jupiter (semitone), Jupiter to Saturn (semitone), and Saturn to the fixed stars or zodiac (one and a half tones). The eighth tone of the scale (also known as "do") completes the full octave. This final tone actually vibrates at twice the frequency of the first "do," but it is so perfect in consonance that it appears to be merely a duplication of the original "do" tone.[34]

Scarantino's interpretation results not in a seven-tone scale, not even a scale really, but rather, just a group of notes with no relation to a scale or to Pythagoras. Further criticism of Scarantino's version of history and acoustics may be cruel. Scarantino is no musician, nor acoustician, nor historian, and perhaps should be spared because she makes no claims to any of these professions. It is therefore even more remarkable when doctors and self-proclaimed music theorists, ethnomusicologists, and musicologists proclaim competence in areas of study in which they are egregiously lacking.

Kay Gardner and Laeh Maggie Garfield

Does naivete or ignorance of technical matters on the part of a composer make for aesthetic errors in composition, or for technical impossibilities? In *Wozzeck*, composer Alban Berg wrote trombone glissandi that were technically impossible. Trombonists "fake" these passages. Many other serious composers have made similar errors, but infrequently. Many New Age healer/composers, though, reveal a lack of technical knowledge in their writing. If Mozart did not know the harmonic series he could not have written for French horn or trumpet. If Stravinsky did not know the harmonic series the *Rite of Spring* would have been devoid of much of the scintillating string writing that helps make it the great piece it is. What are we to assume will be the compositional limitations of Kay Gardner, who writes,

> It is interesting to note that in the past five years, composers of New Age and healing music have simultaneously been scoring their works with a common element of music, *Harmonics*. Without going into the physics of music or a lengthy explanation of harmonics at this time, let me just say that harmonics are the spiritual, mystical element of music. Jonathan Goldman of the New England Sound Healers calls them the Jacob's Ladder between the physical and spiritual. . . . When a fundamental tone is sounded, the physical body will vibrate with it and each succeeding auric body will vibrate to each . . . overtone or harmonic. In the future, harmonics will play an increasingly important part in medical music.[35]

Is Gardner implying that harmonics are a new discovery or that they haven't been a regular feature of sound until recently? A lack of understanding in regard to harmonics is shared by scores of New Age composers and theorists such as Laeh Maggie Garfield (she of the silicondioxide body). "Overtones," she writes, "are resonating multidimensional sounds that originate from a single note. The chanting of Tibetan monks is replete with overtones. Cloistered Catholic monks and nuns sing Gregorian chants, a beautiful, melodic, poetic form of singing containing overtones that echo throughout the chapel and along the corridors of the monastery. The songs serve to clear the mental/emotional planes, thereby permitting greater access to the Source and your own soul."[36]

Cloistered Catholic monks and nuns may indeed sing Gregorian chants, and when they do there will be overtones, but there will occur the same overtones when fifty thousand World Series fans sing "Take Me Out to the Ball Game," during the seventh-inning stretch, only more of them. Garfield suggests that, "Overtones is an incorrect and confusing translation from the German word *Obertone*."[37] Actually "overtone" is a correct term for harmonics above a fundamental. Garfield prefers "uppertones." She writes, "Uppertones is a clever and more accurate word for the whole series of higher tones emanating from a musical note,"[38] but she does not realize in this superfluous coinage that overtones are synonymous with harmonics (except for the enumeration), as well as with the word "partial"; "partial" is synonymous in enumeration as well with "harmonic." This duplicity of meaning (triplicity, actually) may be a trifle confusing, but Garfield raises confusion to an art form by declaring that these words, which mean the same thing, are actually different.

> As an example, when we strike the C-string of a cello or piano, the sound we hear is made up of various tones called partial tones. All the partial tones within a single note are referred to as a compound or complex tone. The lowest partial tone is the fundamental or prime tone. It is the loudest tone of the whole series; therefore we name that string's

sound after its prime tone. All the other partial tones are upper partials or Uppertones.[39]

In addition to Garfield's new coinage of "uppertone," she adds "prime tone," which is her neologism for the fundamental. Garfield also gives a lesson in the difference between quantity and quality. "The psychological or aesthetic characteristics that correspond to the physical characteristics are pitch, loudness, and quality. Studying the theory of overtones offers you an opportunity to understand the link between quantity and quality."[40] Searching through Garfield's book does not result in an explanation of how the theory of overtones will aid in the understanding of even just Laeh Garfield. Unlike Randall McClellan, Garfield does understand that the harmonic series is potentially infinite, but she is enamored of adding confusion to a subject already difficult enough.

> The hertzian number relationship of overtones has a certain mode that is the same for every fundamental note. . . . We call the relationship of hertz-numbers of these partial tones harmonics. Together they create a sound of harmony. In addition to the limits of the audible range, there are limits to our hearing discrimination wherein it becomes impossible to hear the separate overtones. Although the measured hertz interval from partial tone to partial tone is equal, the pitch-interval (the height difference of the partials as we hear them) gets smaller and smaller until we cannot hear the difference anymore.[41]

If Garfield's book, *Sound Medicine,* was read simply for pleasure and/or humor there would be no point in criticizing its all-too-apparent ignorance of acoustics and science. However, though Garfield's science stands out among music-healing books as transparently absurd; her book is read by other music healers, given credence, and even cited as an "important and pragmatic book" by Kay Gardner in *Sounding the Inner Landscape.*[42]

The conclusion of Garfield's chapter on acoustics is nonpareil:

Paul Horn, the flutist, was leaving for the Great Pyramid in Egypt hoping to record inside of it, when he received a phone call. The man on the other end informed him that the inside of the Great Pyramid would yield the note A minus 231. Curious as to how his caller knew he asked if the man had played inside of it. "No," replied the mathematician, "I figured it out from the dimensions." Later inside the pyramid Paul Horn discovered his caller had been absolutely correct.[43]

Until this moment I was not aware that frequency could be negative. Equally surprising is that, "Horn discovered his caller had been absolutely correct." How Horn could know that the anonymous caller was right defies explanation. To test the caller's veracity Horn would have had to have heard the pyramid played (though we are not told how, in fact, one goes about playing the Great Pyramid) and Horn would have had to have had the capacity to *hear* the imaginary pitch "A minus 231". Paul Horn should not be held responsible in any way for Garfield's amusing fantasy.

Mystical Acoustics

R. J. Stewart

R. J. Stewart's metaphysical theories of music are based on secrecy. The body of his book *Music and the Elemental Psyche* contains little acoustical data, but in his fifth appendix, buried deep in the back of his tome, Stewart reveals his secret knowledge. "The proportions of the scale (first, second, third, and so on) are strict mathematical acoustic entities *except in modern music, where they have been adjusted or tempered*" (emphasis mine).[44] In fact, tempered music has strict mathematical acoustic properties, as much as the untempered natural harmonic series. The major difference is the opposite of what Stewart implies. Whereas in equal temperament all identical intervals (such as C to D and D to E) are exactly alike, in the earlier systems and in the natural harmonic series the proportions differ. In the natural harmonic series a major second may have a frequency ratio of 9:8, or 10:9, 12:11, 13:12, or 8:7, just to name some of the most frequently occurring ratios. In equal temperament all major seconds are exactly alike (which is why, of course, it is called equal temperament).

Stewart theorizes that, "In an untempered scale our various notes will be of differing rates of vibration (although called by the same letter of the alphabet) *depending upon the direction by which we approach them.* This important micro-tonal difference is the key to a very ancient method of chanting and playing music, and is still found in the sacred and magical music of the East today as a tradition in which the metaphysical elements or systems are only partly understood."[45]

To be sure, the use of the untempered scale is partly understood by Stewart, who gathers his information, he himself notes, from brief entries in musical dictionaries, and not correctly at that. The harmonic series is no esoteric secret. The notes of the untempered scale are not magic. One need not join a mystical society to bow harmonics on a cello. As for the untempered scale's notes changing "depending upon the direction by which we approach them," this is a proposition that is hair-raising in its implications. If two singers approach the same pitch, one from above (descending) and one from below (ascending), does Stewart mean to say that they will not arrive at the same pitch? They will sing an out-of-tune unison purposefully? This is what he is saying, yet a practice as unpleasant as this has never been, not in any earthly culture, not even Bulgaria. Untempered pitch is not determined by direction, or theory, or anything really. Untempered pitch is natural pitch. It simply is. It is tempered pitch that has to be altered, and even then the alteration is never determined by direction, but by the particular system of temperament in use, so that a pitch approached from either direction by any performer is always in tune at the unison.

Dane Rudhyar

Dane Rudhyar combines a Westernized version of Buddhism with a typical disesteem for Western culture, while still remaining firmly anchored in it. Yet Rudhyar is naive about the application of oriental philosophies to oriental musical systems. "Tonality is a European system," he misinforms in *The Magic of Tone and the Art of Music.*

> Tonality, in the strict sense of the term, is the product of European society. . . . Tonality can be considered the autocratic rule of the king (the tonic). . . . But it is also the power of a bureaucracy that measures and enforces the exact *distances* between all the factors in the whole. Tonality is a system by which the innate pluralism of a society is kept within a definite operative structure . . . sequences of chords under and (through their overtones) around the melodic sequence of tones ensure the feeling of unity. Each melodic tone carries an identifying badge announcing clearly where it belongs, not so much in relation to the tonic as in terms of its place and function in the tonal bureaucracy. . . . This is the ransom of the ideal of universalism. . . . In our pluralistic European music the instinctual psychic power of integration that once was inherent in sequences of tones had to be replaced by the harmonizing impact of chords clearly stating the tonality to which melodic notes belong.[46]

Rudhyar excludes all non-European music from the bane of polarity, the feeling of a dominant pitch. He must be unaware that in Indian music there is a pitch called the "King" pitch, which, of course, functions like the European tonic pitch. If a sociopolitical argument is to be made based upon musical systems, it is not the oriental nor any other non-European culture's music that contains pluralistic concepts in its musical language. Rather, it is *only* Western music that escapes the monarchy of tonality. In a vast number of non-European musical systems, key pitches are referred to as kings, leaders, and gods, while other pitches are labeled as inferior or as servants to the kingly pitches. Since the development of the European equal temperament system, the classical composers of Western music have continuously moved further and further away from the concept of tonic pitches. In the twentieth century composers freed themselves entirely from the concept of dominant tones and created music that purposefully evaded the labeling that still accurately reflects the musical systems of non-European cultures. The school of serialism dictated a technique whereby all twelve pitches of the chromatic scale are absolutely identical in weight and importance, a perfect musical Marxism (and with a similar fate). Polytonal composers like Stravinsky and his followers created music in which several key pitches ruled simultaneously. Neo-Romantic composers such as Sibelius eschewed the rule of any tonal center in favor of rotating leaderships, and the rest of twentieth-century art-music composers are associated with the school aptly named, atonality, in which no tonal center whatsoever exists. It is the twentieth-century composer's denial of a primary status to certain pitches that defines him and was made possible by the adoption four hundred years ago of the pluralistic, equal-temperament system, which allowed composers to modulate freely, no longer servant to the tonic pitch. If Rudhyar, a twentieth-century composer himself, truly believes in the social agenda he describes as being served by an analogous musical system, he should be attacking the musical systems of all people but the serial, atonal, and polytonal composers of twentieth-century Europe.

Rudhyar denies "Archaic peoples" the intellect to "respond to music esthetically. The feeling of what we call a melody probably did not exist in ancient, preclassical Greece or in the Egypt and Chaldea of 3000 B.C."[47] Allotting magical properties to the music of prehistory, Rudhyar manages to sound just like the European straw man he professes to detest when he writes, "Specific inflections and modes of intonation are not melodies, in the traditional European sense, nor are the chants of American Indian corn dances, healing rituals, or other sacred ceremonies."[48] Incapable of melodic invention, in his opinion, non-European people cannot preserve their musical culture as can Westerners.

> When these chants are written down in Western musical notation, the power of the psychism that was their source is totally lost. They become like x-ray photographs, devoid of living flesh. Even when recorded

directly on tape, the chants are no longer psychoactive because nothing that belongs strictly to the life of a culture-whole can retain its psychic power when it is taken away from the place and circumstances in which it fulfilled an organic function. . . . While there are obvious similarities among the "x-ray pictures" of diatonically notated tribal chants and sacred rituals from all over the world, the similarities exist because all peoples belong to the same biological species that has developed in the biosphere of the same planet.[49]

Rudhyar claims that music has psychic parameters that cannot be transferred to paper. Assuming this, then, how can the written notation of classical music be any different, assuming (as Rudhyar correctly does) that even Europeans "belong to the same biological species" as Indians?

If an ethnomusicologist transcribes the Balinese Monkey Chant using the notational system of European classical music, he is not doing damage merely to the "psychic" aspects of the Monkey Chant, he is not doing his job well at all. Western musical notation can only serve to capture the musical intentions of composers who use that system. The system is not better, nor worse, than others; it is merely culture-specific. Good ethnomusicologists are constantly striving to clarify their musical symbology to better capture the music of other cultures. Rudhyar is merely excoriating bad ethnomusicologists for their bad work. But this in no way can imply that a musical system not of European derivation cannot be accurately transcribed. The rules and practices of non-European musics are as specific and highly limited as are those of Europe.

Rudhyar states that notation systems can never capture the essence of music, nor even can a mechanically recorded version succeed. Therefore, musical culture can never be shared outside a country's boundaries. We who cannot afford to go to Bali may just as well throw away our recordings of the splendid Monkey Chant. Further, even attending a live performance of a Beethoven string quartet is rendered meaningless because, after all, the performers are reading their parts from scores. Finally, as Rudhyar is a composer one must ask why he destroys his own musical intentions by putting his music in the form of "x-ray photographs devoid of living flesh" scores and recordings.

Rudhyar says, "The first thing cellist Pablo Casals did every morning was to play a particular work of Bach. . . . A Hindu brahmin would have meditated and intoned the sacred chant gayatri, but the psychic meanings of the gayatri and of a Bach composition are essentially different."[50] Rudhyar's proclamation is naively racist. The Brahmin and Casals have different skin tones, perhaps, but Rudhyar implies that it really is not true that we're all the same species after all.

Common to all species of New Age music commentators, Rudhyar has a lot to say about acoustics and music theory.

> The three components of the diatonic scale—the tonic, dominant and subdominant—are the foundations of the harmono-melodic tonality system. They were also the basis of the Pythagorean scale whose application, at least in its origin, was monodic rather than melodic. Melody comes into music, we can assume, with the popular or folk element. This element had its concentrated appeal in the natural intonation interval of the third—the relationship between the fourth and fifth harmonics of the harmonic series. On the other hand, the Pythagorean third (C to E) apparently was derived from the fifth note of a series of exact fifths (C, G, D, A, E) reduced to the musical space of an octave. The difference between a Pythagorean third and a "natural" third (the 5:4 ratio) could be compared to the difference between the theoretically impersonal relationship of a monk and nun, or between any two members of an ashram, and the personal love of an ordinary man and woman.[51]

The imputation that the "Pythagorean scale" and hence the Greek modes used the tonic, dominant, and subdominant relations of classical Western music is contradicted by the writings of the contemporary Greek writers who described the music of Greece. These "three components of the diatonic scale" are a relatively recent development, and do not pertain to Pythagorean tuning. A Pythagoras-based intonation had to be dropped because of the emerging use of "classical" tonality five hundred years ago; it was replaced with the mean-tone system. Pythagoras-based intonation could not accommodate the music of Europe, as the use of modulation and its chromatic alterations developed in the evolution of the dominant and subdominant key relationships.

Rudhyar's hypothesis about the derivation of the major third from Pythagorean intonation is dead wrong. Rudhyar fails to differentiate between major and minor thirds which, within the mean-tone system, were derived from the intervals between the fourth and fifth and the fifth and sixth harmonic of the harmonic series, and not, as he incorrectly assumes, from Pythagorean intonation.

Many oriental pentatonic systems are tuned exclusively with 3:2 Pythagorean intervalic ratios, though that method was developed independent of Pythagoras. Not knowing this, Rudhyar inadvertently dismisses the folk music of China because it uses Pythagorean tuning. Chinese pentatonic music does not contain the 5:4 third relationship that Rudhyar holds sacrosanct, but rather the third relationship based exactly upon the evil mechanism he describes as Pythagorean. Rudhyar writes:

> Because of the particular kind of musical motion called modulation, and because of the increasing use of the piano or similar instruments with fixed keyboards, a chromatic division of the octave into twelve equal intervals has become the fundamental feature of Western music. The equalized series of octaves and twelve fifths produces a musical space divided into eighty-four equal intervals. This has become for two and a half centuries the materia prima of Western music. This music has spread all over the globe, together with technological products and a personalistic way of life. As we shall see in greater detail in chapter 11, the piano keyboard can be made to represent the entire world of now-usable musical sounds. It can also be considered a symbol of the sociopolitical and ethical organization of theoretically free and equal individuals, without any functional or generic, religious or financial, ideological or characterological differentiation—the organization called democracy.[52]

Equal temperament is not restricted to Europe. Equal temperaments of seven- and five-note scales occur, for example, in Thailand and Africa. Pythagorean intonation is not equal temperament. The Pythagorean fifth does not equal the equal-temperament fifth. When Rudhyar states that equal-temperament consists of twelve equal-tempered fifths he misses the point entirely. Pythagorean intonation consists of a uniform fifth interval throughout seven octaves based upon the natural 3:2 relationship of the second and third harmonic of the harmonic series. In equal temperament it is not the fifth that has equal intervalic ratios, but rather the fifths, sixths, sevenths, seconds, thirds, and fourths, none of which matches exactly any of the intervalic ratios of the first sixteen harmonics of the harmonic series, with the exception of the octave.

The assumption that "the piano keyboard can be made to represent the entire world of now-usable musical sounds" is absurdly erroneous. The piano is a marvellous instrument with an extraordinary range, but it is technically incapable of capturing the totality of Western musical expression for a number of reasons, the two most obvious being its inability to carry out the glissando and the crescendo. No matter the intent of the pianist, once the hammer strikes a key the dynamic has nowhere to go but down. An instrument such as the oboe, with the range of barely two octaves, is able to create beautiful music on a single swelling pitch that the pianist can listen to only in admiring envy. Furthermore, the equal-temperament system developed during the autocratic period in Europe, not the democratic period in America. Rudhyar's claim for connection between democracy and equal temperament is ahistorical. He cannot possibly cite the existence of a single democracy in the entire Western world concurrent with Bach's composition of the "Well-Tempered Clavier." And equating democracy with equal temperament completely contradicts Rudhyar's earlier assertion that Western music is hopelessly mired in the concept of monarchy. Possibly Rudhyar realized his earlier metaphor was nonsensical. However, it would be wise for him to recall the ahistoricity of his new metaphor.

That the piano is an obstacle to many New Age music theoreticians' understanding Pythagoras and music of other cultures should not be over-looked. A New Age music theorist whose background is piano often becomes confused when delving into the world of non-Western music, in which the piano's restricted pitches can not fully capture the actual pitches of the foreign culture's music.

Don Campbell

Don Campbell discusses the improvisatory techniques that he used on a piano-forte while accompanying a dance company; in doing so, reveals a lack of understanding regarding temperaments and scales.

> I disciplined myself to improvise for a week at a time on each Grego-rian mode, and I began to hear beyond the chordal structure I had learned in eighteenth-century counterpoint. As I spent those hours in *lydian* and *phrygian* modes, I also began to sense different body pos-tures and moods. What at first seemed to be a monotonous exercise turned into a state of mind where many new musical ideas could emerge. . . . I wondered if it was my imagination or if there was some truth about the transformative power in the great Pythagorian modes and Greek temperaments. My ear had previously been able to identify the modes, but I had never before spent enough time with them to hear the power of which the ancients spoke.[53]

Campbell could not have learned about the value of "the great Pythagorean modes and Greek temperaments" on a piano-forte, which is tuned in equal-tempered intervals (or even on his flute). As for the "Greek temperaments," if he knows what they sound like he is unique today, as there was no information in Pythagoras or indeed any music commenta-tor during the period of the use of the true Greek modes that explained, beyond poetic metaphor, what the tunings were. Unfortunately, it may be that Campbell is making the freshman music major mistake of confusing the church modes of European derivation with the authentic Greek modes of millennia past. The only similarity between the two is the names. "lydian" mode nowadays refers to the church mode of that name, a mode used in singing Gregorian chant. The Greek "Lydian" mode is lost forever. Greek modes were not tuned using Pythagorean temperament, and there is no such thing as the Pythagorean modes. This is an invention of Campbell's. What Campbell actually did was play equal-tempered diatonic scales beginning on different white keys of the piano, without the employment of accidentals.

What is it about the natural harmonic series and equal temperament that confuses so many New Age music theorists? Geoffrey Hodson in his book *Music Forms* relies on Gordon Kingsley for music theory expertise. In Kingsley's introduction to Hodson's "Eight Compositions Clairvoyantly Observed," Kingsley writes,

> Every scale whose series of notes designate a particular "key" is a small fraction out of tune, purposely made so in order that other keys may not suffer, but may be sufficiently well in tune for all workable purposes.
>
> In the days of Bach this was not the case. A few of the keys—those most often employed—were tuned in perfect pitch [*sic*] with the result that the remainder were so lamentably out of tune that musicians rarely, if ever, used them. But Bach was opposed to this procedure. He felt, and rightly, that each key has its own especial beauties, C major has basic solidity, C minor is sombre, D-flat major is mellifluous, C-sharp minor—its relative—is mystical, and so on. Each key might be likened to one of the component colours in the spectrum with the resultant white light, the blending of them all.[54]

No, no, no. This is the opposite of the truth. Where Kingsley is not completely wrong, he is completely confused. The mean-tone system, the tuning system since the sixteenth century, was not "tuned in perfect pitch," nor was it an untempered natural scale. The natural harmonic series had not been employed in Europe for over a millennium (in sacred and art music). Bach supported equal temperament (though really only a close approximation) not because "each key has its own especial beauties," but because he desired to modulate to diverse keys within a piece impossible in the mean-tone system. Quite the reverse of Kingsley's claims, equal temperament does away with the individuality of different keys, creating a system of intonation in which the only acoustically natural interval is the octave. Bach was not interested in preserving the individuality of keys as was, perforce, the result of the mean-tone system, but rather in destroying the individuality of the keys in order to better express his complex harmonic modulations.

In the mean-tone system enharmonically equivalent tones such as G♯ and A♭ were extremely different pitches, the A♭ being nearly a quarter tone higher than the G♯. Without equal temperament, complicated modulations wherein the A♭ of one section becomes reinterpreted as a G♯ in the next were impossible. Goodbye to Beethoven and all the composers who follow him. As for Bach, the vast majority of his pieces become unplayable, and unlistenable. In the Courante from his second partita, the lowest voice in the third measure contains the following pitches: G, then A♭, then F♯. In mean-tone temperament the interval between A♭ and F♯ would be excruciating. The A-natural that follows (in the inner voice) adds aural injury to wolftone insult.

In 1821 Beethoven composed his Piano Sonata in A♭, opus 110. Its opening movement, a work of sublime beauty, pivots on the modulation from A-flat major to E major. This modulation, impossible in the mean-tone system, is a vindication of the equal-temperament system, a system in which all keys become ciphers of one another. The "especial beauties" of each key are replaced with the beauty of relations. C major no longer can mean anything in particular, but must rely on the context in which it is used. How is it that New Age music theorists see (I eschew using the word "hear" in place of "see" here, as it would be misleading) vast differences between keys in which the intervals between all pitches are identical, regardless of the key? While the mean-tone system was in use there were legitimate differences (though these were not uniform because different instruments were tuned differently), and a clear case could be made for hearing the keys differently, but now such arguments are nonsense.

Even more puzzling, what is the reason for the great disesteem New Age music theorists purport to hold for equal temperament? I say purport because though they attack it they themselves do not restrain themselves from using it. Donald Campbell in *The Roar of Silence* expresses immense displeasure with equal temperament and the evolution of Western harmony.

> Our Western modes slowly fell into disuse after the year 1600 when the didactic major scale (inappropriately labeled "happy" by music teachers) and minor scale (similarly misnamed "sad") became the usual standard for musical expression. We seemed to lose some of the range and subtlety of emotions available to the ancients by the very strange idea that there is "happy" music and "sad" music. Fortunately, through the educational innovation and intuitive awareness of Hungarian composer Zoltan Kodaly and German composer Carl Orff, American and British children are again being richly taught the pentatonic (five note) scales and ancient modes.[55]

Setting aside arguments about Campbell's belief that American and British children are being "richly" taught ancient modes, I wonder why Campbell's own New Age compositions do not reflect his displeasure with Western equal temperament. Campbell's "Crystal Meditations" is a synthesized, electronic piece and if Campbell were sincerely displeased with the Western system of equal temperament he need not have employed it. As he realizes his compositions with the use of a synthesizer, Campbell has the opportunity to use any temperament system he wishes. Synthesizers can be programmed to realize in mean-tone intonation, Pythagorean or just intonation, or totally invented intonations. A composer who truly wishes to compose music outside the confines of the equal-temperament system has no obstacle to so doing thanks to computer realization. Nevertheless, not Campbell nor any music healer who shares Campbell's professed disdain for the equal-temperament system uses any intonation system but equal temperament for their New Age compositions. I question the sincerity of all New Age music healer/composers who clamor against equal temperament and yet choose to compose exclusively in it. No one is holding a gun to Donald Campbell's head, forcing him to use equal temperament. There have been many composers who utilized other temperament systems and/or created their own. Harry Partch is one of the most famous exemplars.

Classical music's use of major and minor keys carry no such simplistic distinctions such as happy and sad. Classical music is highly subjective. Even a programmatic piece such as the "Marcia Funebre" from Beethoven's Opus 26 is ambiguous. Is it funereal? What is the meaning of the transition at the end to major? If it is death, why does the sonata continue after the funeral march? Beethoven had no desire to restrict our contemplation of Opus 26 to his own motivations in composing it. His title may be viewed as his "opinion," or, perhaps, a rhetorical device: an argument. Whether the piece is about death, or rebirth, or pride, or whatever, is really not Beethoven's business; it is ours.[56]

If Campbell hears major and minor as happy and sad, this is his limitation, not classical music's. Furthermore, Campbell's assertion that music teachers label major and minor scales as happy and sad, followed by the statement "we seemed to lose some of the range and subtlety of emotions available to the ancients," implies that these erroneous music teachers have actually destroyed Western music. Does Beethoven lack range and subtlety? Does Mozart? Palestrina? Have music teachers corrupted their messages, or does Campbell mean that Beethoven never did express "subtlety" and never had range? Was Brahms a shallow composer or are we incapable, because of our inept music teachers, of appreciating his work? Not incidentally, it is likely that bad teachers are not a recent development on this planet and the "ancients" had their share of them.

Kay Gardner

Kay Gardner, who is fond of espousing oriental music philosophy and attacking Western art music's acoustic foundations writes,

In our western music, we work with fewer than 100 scales, whereas in South India there are more than 5000 different scales. Granted that Indian music includes quarter tones and micro-tones, but still it shows that western music is very limited and limiting. In India there are ragas for all times of day, ragas to accompany all kinds of daily activities and ragas which reflect and accompany bodily functions.

We also must turn to old and new tuning systems other than the chaotic equal-temperament with which we have been saddled almost exclusively since the invention of the piano. By turning away from pure intervals and the resulting mix of harmonics, we have ignored the very scales which ancient and medieval medical practitioners found so effective.[57]

Like Campbell, Gardner completely contradicts her written philosophy with her music. She records musical pieces that she labels authentic Indian ragas, that are neither Indian nor ragas nor does she even bother to have her instrumentalists employ the Indian twenty-two *sruti* temperament system. Incredibly, Gardner employs (you guessed it) equal temperament, which is incompatible with Indian music. One cannot play authentic Indian ragas using European equal temperament. But not only does she play these "ragas" in equal temperament, she solemnly announces over the fake raga that she is playing an authentic Indian raga in her recent release, *Sounding the Inner Landscape*.[58] In addition to her misinformation about her raga, Gardner chooses to use a majority of European instruments that have been refined for hundreds of years to perform in equal temperament. Why does Gardner not use authentic Indian music or the intonation system of authentic Indian music when she performs music she claims is authentically Indian? Is her point that: Indian music's beautiful and unique intonation system can be replaced by a handful of Americans on mostly Western instruments playing simple melodic and harmonic pseudo-ragas in equal temperament? In *Sounding the Inner Landscape*, Gardner not only misrepresents Indian music, but desecrates the traditional musics of other cultures as well. In a section in which she professes to demonstrate the "Greek" modes (by which she really means the church modes) Gardner fails to accomplish even an accurate demonstration of the church modes. Her musicians perform the wrong modes apparently unaware that the ostinato bass that pervades the music is changing the tonal center. There are unintentionally comic moments (for those who know the Church modes) when intervals and melodies prove irreconcilable with her voice-over labeling.

In "Processional" from *A Rainbow Path*,[59] a recording of Kay Gardner's music based on the "eight" (*sic*) chakras, she claims to use the *saraswati* raga in C, the same raga she uses in *Sounding the Inner Landscape*. The piece is not a "*saraswati* raga in C." It is possible that Gardner's misidentification is but a remnant of the influence of a nineteenth-century text in which C. R. Day, an ethnomusicologically illiterate Englishman, Anglicized five hundred ragas as his hobby while serving in the British army in colonial India. Unfortunately, his distortions have been passed on unchecked in numerous pseudo-ethnomusicological works. His *Music and Musical Instruments of Southern India and the Deccan* was published first in 1891 with the promise that the 750 copies would remain unique. But in 1974 its publisher unwisely reprinted it. Day realized that the Indian scale has twenty-two *srutis* and he notes their actual frequencies early in his treatise, but then, in typical chauvinist, imperialist fashion, he lists hundreds of Indian ragas using *only* the Western, equal-tempered pitch symbols, including the "Sarasrati-Manohari," which he begins on C.[60]

Randall McClellan lists exercises in his book *The Healing Forces of Music* for extending the vocal range by singing what he claims to be the pitches of the Indian raga tonal system. But, like Gardner, McClellan ignores the actual Indian classical music tonal system of twenty-two *srutis* and shows a chart in which the Western solfeggio symbols are equated with the Indian pitch names.[61] Those who follow McClellan's "Indian" vocal exercises are just using Indian names for Western solfeggio. One might as well serve Kentucky Fried Chicken and tell your diners that it is Roghan Josh.

These music healers' "Indian" musical practices are reminiscent of the chauvinistic attitude the British took in regard to Indian music in previous centuries. Curt Sachs in *The Wellsprings of Music* describes how

an English High Court judge in Calcutta, William Jones, had in 1784 written *On the musical modes of the Hindoos.* . . . When he quotes his main collector, an English musician in India, as saying that he had had no small trouble in setting the native tunes in a regular (!) "tempo" (he means rhythm), we cannot accept them without reserve and distrust. How the "regularization" was done can indeed be seen from the neat notation of a children's prayer heard in Malabar. . . . The same piece . . . later recorded on an Edison cylinder, found its way to the Phonographic Archives of Berlin, and was published in 1904. The recorded original is sung, as many children's songs of India, in the typical, charming *triputa* rhythm of seven beats or 4 + 3 in the measure.[62]

Sachs proceeds to transcribe, correctly, the song in 7/4, lamenting that the actual music "was too strong a medicine for the good musician from England. And so it came to pass that his 'regularized' version proceeded in the most insipid, hobbling, and banal six-eight."[63]

Kay Gardner's attitude toward Indian music is no different than that of the eighteenth-century British chauvinist. Oblivious to the unique beauty of Indian music, Gardner performs the same regularization—mutilation, really—transmogrifying the *saraswati* raga into an insipid, hobbling, and banal 4/4 simulacrum. Too often, and with saccharine results, do New Age music composers shoehorn Indian music into the Western equal-temperament system. There is no correspondence between the C-major diatonic scale of the West and the seven pitches used in a specific raga. The twenty-two *sruti* system does not fit a piano or a bassoon; and without the twenty-two *sruti* system, Indian music cannot be real Indian music.

Undertones

John Beaulieu

In *Music and Sound in the Healing Arts* John Beaulieu describes a "descending series" of harmonics.[64] But this "descending series" is not logarithmically constructed. It is a fiction, unnatural, and meaningless both musically and acoustically. Of the pitches shown over or under a theoretical C string, only the octave C's occur at a node. His "descending series" tones are not separated by whole number-ratios, a rudimentary prerequisite of pitches related to each other in a harmonic series. If they are not related by whole number ratios it serves no purpose to label them a "harmonic series," as they simply are not a "harmonic series."

Dane Rudhyar

Beaulieu is not alone in this notion of a "subharmonic series," sharing it with other New Age music theorists, including Joscelyn Godwin and Dane Rudhyar, who in *The Magic of Tone and the Art of Music* displays the same meaningless series.[65] Perhaps they are following the musings of the American composer Henry Cowell. Cowell used the "descending harmonic series" as a musical device no different than Schumann's use of the name of his friend, Neil Gade, in a musical work in which the pitches G, A, D, and E are utilized as melodic material. Schumann did not claim that Gade's name had acoustical meaning, nor did Cowell ever attempt to present evidence that his "descending harmonic series" was anything other than an artificial method for creating a melody.

But Rudhyar attempts a scientific, though hopeless, defense of the "descending series," writing,

> This relationship can be demonstrated audibly using a monochord, the
> didactic instrument of Pythagoras's teachings. If one plucks succes-

sively the entire string of the monochord, then one half of it, one third, one fourth, one fifth, and so on, one hears an *ascending* series of harmonics; these are explained by the physical fact that when the string as a whole is plucked it not only vibrates as a whole, but its aliquot parts also vibrate—thus the vibrations of half of the string, a third, a quarter, and a fifth are also perceptible, at least in theory.

If, on the other hand, the hand plucks one inch of the monochord's string, then two inches, three inches, four, five, and six inches, and so on, a *descending* progression of sounds is produced, which gives the hearer a symbolic experience of the path followed by the descent of creative and willful Sound. It is only a symbolic experience, because no part of a descending series of harmonics is audible. What seem to be "undertones" are combination tones (or resulting tones). These are complex auditory phenomena that acousticians consider to be subjective, in the sense that they are apparently produced in the inner ear because of the way the 25,000 extremely delicate hair cells of the cochlea vibrate.[66]

So much wrong, so little space to explain. First, "no part of a descending series of harmonics is audible," because no descending series of harmonics exists. Second, "undertones" are not combination tones. Combination tones (both additive and subtractive) are created by the differences between two pitches, not as just some subjective byproduct of a nonsensical theory. The "descending series" does not contain any relationship to real harmonic or physiological processes. Confusing "undertones" with subtraction tones is evidence of a misunderstanding of acoustics. The contention that "the vibrations of half of the string, a third, a quarter, and a fifth are also perceptible, at least in theory," is further evidence of confusion. It is not "theory," it is demonstrable fact. The Pythagorean monochord theory (inaccurately described by Rudhyar) is easily demonstrated by the simple method described by Pythagoras. There is no string or vibrating body that can duplicate the pitches of the misnamed "descending harmonic series." Rudhyar misleads the reader by describing a process in which it is inferred that this "descending series" is produced. Following the directions in his book, no "descending harmonic series" will be produced.

Joscelyn Godwin

Joscelyn Godwin's *Harmonies of Heaven and Earth* focuses more on the celestial than the mundane. His chapter on the harmonic series deals less with the acoustic principles than with his special symbolic interpretations. The seventh, eleventh, thirteenth, and fourteenth harmonics represent "evil in the world." He says, "To sound the seventh is simply to bring this tendency out into the open. Yet even when it is resolved, the resolution can never be final, for the chord to which it resolves will also contain its own seventh harmonic, its own discontent, like the seed of evil and disharmony present in every being."[67]

Godwin's book is an excellent resource for demonstrating the absurdity of trying to assign universal archetypes to scales, pitches, intervals, and so on, in that Godwin attempts an encyclopedic collection of various hermetic interpretations of secret music teachings. He includes more than a dozen different astrological tone zodiacs, whose differences at least imply originality on behalf of their creators. Godwin fails to draw the conclusion from all this conflicting evidence that the very concept of a tone zodiac is valueless and instead encourages his reader, in the words of P. D. Ouspensky, to "start again. You must make a new beginning. You must reconstruct everything for yourselves—from the very beginning."[68] Very well then, let us take Godwin's advice and begin again.

Tibetan Bowls and Chladni Plates

Steven Halpern

All tones (with the exception of the sine tone) produce harmonics, and these harmonics have frequencies, in simple whole-number ratios to the fundamental. However, certain sound sources produce inharmonic upper partials, most notably, bells. Thus bells produce their peculiar (to them) clanking sounds and charm. The unique feature of bells escapes Steven Halpern, who in a 1988 lecture complained that critics found his Tibetan bowl piece boring. He could not understand why his piece, which he played on an equal-tempered Fender-Rhodes electric piano (which is built in Western tradition to suppress any inharmonic partials) failed to please. During the lecture Halpern produced and played a Tibetan prayer bowl to demonstrate the similarity. As Halpern claims to have hearing superior to all other human beings it is odd that he did not notice the vast difference between the scintillating sound of the Tibetan bowl and the bland, lifeless, electronic simulacrum he used as the vehicle for his Tibetan bowl piece.

This is my version of Tibetan bowls played on a keyboard. The instrument is a Fender Rhodes electric piano, and you hear the phasing in the sound, the little vibrato. Most of the reviewers and critics over the years, typically drinking 5 cups of coffee and coke (both varieties), can't slow down enough to hear what's happening with this music, which is really also a psychotechnology. So that's one aspect I wanted to share with you. . . . I was attracted to an instrument that I first heard in my head, before it was invented, and then when it was invented I bought one, called the Fender Rhodes electric piano. There's no synthesizer yet that does quite what that one does. It's essentially as if you have a string of eighty-eight tuning forks that you could play with your fingers. And for those of you who are musicians (when I was a professional musician playing trumpet and guitar, quite professionally and quite well); this is, however, music that doesn't work right or well on trumpet or electric guitar or bass. So there is an instrument choice. Oboe, for most people, does not work for relaxation. It's like sitting on a thumb tack. Sure, you can relax sitting on a thumb tack. There are people who sleep on nails. But why bother? Why not just use flute or electric piano or harp or something that works so much more easily?[69]

There are altogether too many fallacies in the preceding quote to enumerate, but a few should be addressed. First, the Fender Rhodes, if it did play like a "string of eighty-eight tuning forks," would be not so unique that "no synthesizer" could duplicate this feat, as all synthesizers are capable of producing sine tones. Second, the "little vibrato" in a Fender Rhodes is not caused by phasing, but by amplitude modulation. Phasing can create amplitude modulation, but the reverse is not true. Halpern's use of amplitude modulation is omnipresent in his music.

> Sometimes this is simply a function of the stereo vibrato of my instrument; sometimes it is the function of slightly more elaborate preparations; and sometimes what we hear on the tape when we play it back surprises all of us! In any event, from the time that I began working with this music, I knew intuitively that what has subsequently been described as "the Halpern Effect" owes much to these ancient roots.[70]

This "Halpern Effect," as Halpern modestly labels it, is in actuality nothing more than pressing the vibrato button on his Fender Rhodes and turning a control that determines the extent of the vibrato to near maximum. Every Fender Rhodes has this capability, as do nearly all electronic keyboard instruments made. On a Roland-brand electric piano the "Halpern Effect" is created by pressing a button (one of six) labeled "VIB" (for vibrato). To determine the rate (amplitude modulations per second) and depth (dynamic level of the amplitude modulation) one adjusts the rate and depth controls to the right of the VIB button. True vibrato, as in the case of the string player's technique, is not amplitude modulation, but a slight raising and lowering of frequency. On the Roland this can be done by playing with the pitch control on the far right of the instrument. The "Halpern Effect" as evident on *Spectrum Suite* is amplitude modulation. Notwithstanding Halpern's claim to "the Halpern Effect," Halpern did not invent the vibrato button or have anything to do with the technology behind electronic vibrato; nor was he the first nor will he be the last to make use of this much-overused, trite sound effect. His claim that the vibrato in his pieces is produced by elaborate preparations or mysterious unknown forces is simply bomphilogy.

Perhaps Halpern discovered the "Halpern Effect" in his laboratory . . . or lavatory.

> Sometimes I've found terrific background drone tones for chanting and vocal improvisation in the most unlikely places. The overhead fans in bathrooms are one such example. I can recall at least one time when I was visiting at a friend's house and went to use their bathroom, only to remain there to sing. After several extra moments had elapsed, my host would usually come rushing up to the door, exclaiming, "We wondered what happened to you!" I tell them, and marvel at their disbelief. "Oh, *that* ugly noise . . . ?" they say. "Musician's license," I tell them. "It's not every day that one finds a perfect fifth interval being generated by household pleasantries, and one takes 'em where one can."[71]

A large portion of all of Halpern's lectures and books is devoted to the work of Hans Jenny. To Jenny's photographs of Chladni figures, Halpern imparts a mystical significance. Helmholtz, in *On the Sensations of Tone,* scientifically explains the production of Chladni figures and shows their relationship to his inharmonic partials.[72] (Thus two great mysteries for Halpern—why the critics find his Tibetan bowl piece boring, and what significance there is in a six-pointed star turning into a circle on metallic plates—can both be satisfactorily answered in one section of one chapter in Helmholtz's essential tome.)

Peter Guy Manners

Peter Guy Manners has built an entire music-healing industry on the basis of his attraction to the Chladni plates. He writes about his "experimental method":

In attempting to observe the phenomena of vibration one repeatedly feels a spontaneous urge to make the processes visible and to provide occular evidence of their nature, for it is obvious that by virtue of the abundance, clarity and conscious nature of the information communicated by the eye, our mode of observation must be visual. However great the power of the ear to stir the emotions, however wide-ranging the information it receives, particularly through language, the sense of hearing cannot attain the clarity of consciousness which is native to the sight. . . .

Special mention may be made of E. F. P. Chladni (1756–1827), who discovered the sonorous figures named after him while he was investigating Lichen figures. With a violin bow he stroked metal plates sprinkled with powder and was thus able to make the vibration patterns visible. The vibratory movement caused the powder to move from the antinodes to the nodal lines, and Chladni was thus able to lay down the principles of acoustics (e.g. die Akustik 1802).[73]

As great a scientist as Chladni was (he was the first to propose the extraterrestrial origin of meteorites), he did not "lay down the principles of acoustics." What he discovered in regard his plates was the physical manifestation of nodes in two-dimensional vibrating bodies. New Age music healers fail to understand that Chladni was not satisfied with simply noting the manifestations, but rather used the phenomenon to explore questions of acoustical science.

Manners observes, "It would be really true to say that one can hear what one sees and that one can see what one hears."[74] But he also asserts an opposite view: "Now among all our sense perceptions sound is unique in making itself susceptible in two quite different ways, via the ear, as a direct sense experience and via the eye potentially by the senses of touch and of movement. In the form of certain mechanical movements such as those of a string or a tuning fork, hence the spectator as soon as he begins to investigate acoustic phenomena scientifically finds himself in a unique position."[75]

The above quote captures in two sentences, if sentences they be, Manners' preposterous thought processes. If "sound is unique in making itself susceptible . . . via the ear . . . and via the eye," then sight is also unique in being capable of susceptibility by the ear and the eye. Manners' assertion is inherently self-contradictory. And this is Manners at his most intelligible. Manners also writes,

> In all other fields of perception with the exception of the purely mechanical process the transition to non-stereoscopic colourless observation had the effect that the world consciousness simply seemed to exist, leaving the ensuing hiatus to be filled in by a pattern of imagined kinematic happenings. For example colour of ether vibrations, heat by molecular movements, not so in the sphere of acoustics for here a part of the entire event on account of its genuine kinetic character remains a constant actual observation. In consequence the science of acoustics became for the scientific mind of man a model of the required division between the subjective that is for scientific consideration, and the objective, that is the purely kinematic, part of observation. The field of oral perception seemed to justify the procedure of collecting a mass of phenomena stripped of all its experience by man's soul in meeting them in a purely abstract concept of sound.[76]

Manners indeed has only an abstract concept of sound. He has no concept of acoustics and is comically illiterate in regard that science. In "Cymatics and Its Integrating Phenomenon," Manners writes, "Hans Holt showed that tones which to our ears seemed to have a clear and defined pitch may be split up in a series of resonators into a number of different tones. . . . Hans Holt further showed that the particular series of overtones into which a tone can be resolved is responsible for the colour of that tone as a whole."[77]

Manners has learned his acoustics by ear, and a very bad ear at that, as he has confused Helmholtz with an imaginary Hans Holt. Obviously, Helmholtz's name came up in conversation and Manners did not hear correctly, rendering Helmholtz as "Hans Holt." Can one take seriously acoustical theorizing by a man completely unfamiliar with Helmholtz? "Hans Holt"? This is pitiful testimony to Manners's acoustic expertise or lack thereof.

Strangely, Manners seems to know medicine no better than acoustics despite credentials that state he is a medical doctor. Manners states that the brain is "electrically positive." All other "body tissues" are "electrically negative."[78] "The electricity in our bodies is self-generated and starts with our first breath—perhaps even in the womb."[79] Manners's acoustical and medical opinions are cited in even the least eccentric New Age music healers' works.

David Tame, and Halpern and Savary

The study of inharmonic partials is a most difficult area in the science of acoustics. It is not surprising that most standard acoustics texts give short shrift to this consternating discipline. When New Age music theoreticians attempt to delve into the subject, lacking the prerequisite knowledge of the simpler harmonic series, their writing becomes fanciful, even mythic. David Tame in *The Secret Power of Music* writes, "Ernst Chladni, a German physicist, developed what became known as Chladni plates around 1800. These violin-shaped metal plates are able to render visible the kind of vibrations which are natural to violins. The plates are evenly covered with sand, and a bow then drawn across certain points on the edge of the plate. The result is that the sand moves quickly into the pattern of the waves of vibration produced on the plate."[80]

Tame seems never to have seen a Chladni plate if he really believes they are "violin-shaped," as they are in no way "violin-shaped," nor do they move "into the pattern of the waves of the vibration," but rather into symmetrical, predictable (see Helmholtz) forms based on half-wave lengths.

Tame is not alone in his confusion about the Chladni plates. Where he imagines they are violin shaped, Halpern and Savary make the mistake that Chladni plates are not bowed, but rather respond to a nearby violinist, as they report that Chladni "scattered sand on steel discs and observed the changing sand patterns produced by playing different notes on a violin. . . . It is quite possible . . . that the geometrical and vortical forms appearing on Dr. Jenny's discs do so because they symbolically represent an underlying order of the physical universe and human consciousness."[81]

The basic confusion in the music healer's fictions about Chladni plates is their failure to use Chladni's own work, or even Helmholtz's reliable text. It is like a game of telephone in which a message is whispered to one person who subsequently whispers said message to the next player, and so forth, until finally, the last person to receive the message recites what is usually a humorously distorted version of the original. Manners, Tame, and Halpern and Savary relate the Chladni experiments in just this fashion. In actuality, the plates are metal discs (or squares, or other geometric shapes). They are not violin-shaped; rather, they are set in motion with a violin bow (or cello bow). Playing a violin next to the Chladni plates, as Halpern and Savary misconstrue, will produce no discernible effect upon the Chladni plates. One does not play different pitches on any instrument in the vicinity of the plate, one plays the plate itself.

According to Halpern and Savary, "If sand particles can arrange themselves in the presence of pure musical vibrations, is it not possible that musical vibrations, made by musical instruments or our own voices, can have an effect on how the cells of our body are arranged?"[82] The sand particles do not "arrange themselves," they simply bounce around, falling randomly until they land on a part of the Chladni plate (the node) that is not vibrating. When my daughter was one and a half she used to pound on her dinner tray and watch rice puffs bounce around until the puffs had all bounced off the tray onto the floor. Halpern and Savary would say that the rice puffs had "rearranged themselves" onto the floor. The rice puffs simply bounced around randomly until my child (analogous to the standing wave on the Chladni plate) could not affect them anymore. Tame also invokes the Chladni plates in connection with New Age philosopher Lyall Watson. Not surprisingly, Tame finds the plates significant.

The Chladni plates *are* attractive. My daughter has enjoyed playing with them at Philadelphia's Franklin Institute, but what is the fuss about? "Through Jenny's apparatus," writes Tame about another nonfunctional follower of Chladni, "it is possible literally to see what one is hearing."[83] This is no more so than watching the patterns of Beethoven's Ninth Symphony on an oscilloscope is the same as hearing it.

According to Tame, "Other researchers have found a relationship between sound frequencies and various physical—even *notational* shapes. For example, 540 vs. 300 frequency cycles per second [*sic*] displayed on an oscilloscope produces a minor seventh shape."[84] As the oscilloscope is constructed to produce a visual analogy of sound, it is not unfair to ask if the preceding quote means anything other than: an oscilloscope can be observed doing what it was built to do. In fact, if an oscilloscope does not produce a visual representation of a frequency as it was built to do, then it is probably just not plugged in.

Tame shares a basic misunderstanding with many other New Age theorists, videlicit: that the logarithmic qualities of sound, the principles and laws of acoustics, are news, or newsworthy, in and of themselves. There is no denying that acoustics is a subfield of physics, nor that basic universal mathematical principles apply to it; what of it? The ratios of the harmonic series are simple number ratios and anyone can draw any connections they wish from them. Choosing certain numbers and assigning them magical properties is easy, but ultimately nugatory. Tame writes,

> There are in particular a number of fundamental occurrences in nature of the number seven. There are seven rows in the periodic table of elements. A slightly different way of ordering the elements is to give the two rare-earth series basically their own rows in the table, but still we find that this gives us seven rows of *stable* elements. . . . All this is highly suggestive of the possibility that the seven rows of elements rep-

resent the categories of elements which embody the frequencies and properties of each of the seven major Tones. (The number seven also occurs within the human anatomy, in such things as the seven major hormonal glands and the seven ventricles or cavities of the skull.)[85]

Might one counter that the first four octaves of the harmonic series contain sixteen partials, and this coincides with the number of teeth in the lower jaw of the average adult Caucasian male? It is easy to play with numbers and create apparent relationships where there really are no relationships. Defending the number of pitches in the Western diatonic scale as being determined or related to the number of rows on the chart of the known elements is as easy and meaningless as drawing a parallels between the harmonic series and teeth. Tame writes,

> The seven colours of the rainbow are violet, indigo, blue, green, yellow, orange and red. These, and the entire span of the spectrum, are usually depicted in a straight line, one colour blending into the other from violet at one end to red at the other. Yet it is more revealing, and closer to the truth behind all things, to position the colours around the circumference of a circle. It is then possible to see how the solar-spectrum relates to the circle of the zodiac, which in itself is expressive of the total number of twelve tones.[86]

Ignoring the impossibility of turning seven colors into the twelve signs of the zodiac, could I not suggest that the Fourteenth Amendment to the Constitution (citizenship rights not to be abridged), which was ratified in 1868, is amazing, and perhaps significant in regard to the fact that in 1868 a standard tuning fork of the United States, as registered at Chickering's in New York City, produced an A of 451.9 Hz, and that if we calculate C from that A, and then calculate the fourteenth partial above that C of 133.4 Hz, we find that the fourteenth partial is 1868 Hz? Let us review the amazing phenomenon just revealed: (1) The pitch of A in 1868 was

451.9 Hz; (2) the pitch of C of 133.4 Hz is derived from the pitch A of 451.9 Hz; (3) the fourteenth partial of C (133.4 Hz) is 1868 Hz; (4) the Fourteenth Amendment to the Constitution was ratified in 1868.

So, what does this mean: that the amendments to the U.S. Constitution depend on the frequency of "A" during a constitutional convention; or that as music can be reduced to mathematical symbols, any capable acoustician can invent "significance" for any acoustical phenomenon and that even untrained "music theorists" can see meaning behind the simple mathematical truisms of music and acoustics? The world is filled with mathematical coincidences. One can infer mystical meanings in Pythagoras or the pyramids, and the New Age has accumulated attractive fables and myths about acoustics and medicine. Yet, would one want to trust one's health to a music healer whose theories are based upon incorrect assumptions about acoustics? And if the music healer is not only unfamiliar with acoustics, but invents nonsensical acoustic theories as the basis for his healing abilities, can one believe that the rest of his contentions are true? Should we trust music healers who are touting anti-acoustic principles as verifiable reality, while at the same time acknowledging acoustics as the principle with which they have constructed their theories? Their errors are not errors of insignificance. They attest to a deep misconception about how sound works, and hence music healers, through their own testimony, often disqualify themselves from the role they presumptuously assume.

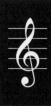

6. Vibrations: Right Effort

Resonance

The term *resonance* has been borrowed from the field of acoustics by writers in every discipline, none more so than the New Age music healer. The acoustical phenomenon of resonance can be briefly and simply explained. A body that is vibrating periodically pushes the air (or other medium) around it, creating waves with the same "frequency" of the vibrating sound source. As the wave travels, it loses energy; but if there is in the vicinity of the original sound source, another elastic object with the same frequency or multiple thereof and the wave front is strong enough, it can cause this second sound source to begin vibrating periodically. This phenomenon is also known as sympathetic vibration.

Many instruments capitalize upon this phenomenon, for example, various stringed instruments employ sympathetic strings. Sympathetic strings are neither plucked nor bowed, but are set in motion by sympathetic vibration. The Indian sitar has twelve or thirteen sympathetic strings beneath the three to seven strings actively used by the instrumentalist. If the performer plays a pitch of 200 Hz (these and the following frequencies are not actual frequencies, but used for the sake of simplicity) and there are three sympathetic strings pitched at 200 Hz, 600 Hz, and 800 Hz, these three strings will resonate. A sympathetic string of 280 Hz will not resonate because it is neither the same frequency, nor a harmonic of the original sound source. When playing a raga on a sitar, sympathetic strings are set in motion and as the performer cannot stop their vibration, a drone (a persistent sonority) is caused. Some Western instruments of the past were built with sympathetic strings, but because Western music modulates within a piece and uses numerous harmonies even when not modulating, these sympathetic strings have been abandoned. In Indian classical music the harmony (and this is applying a Western label that is not quite appropriate) is static, and thus the drone does not interfere with the music, but, like instruments of all cultures, instead, is an integral part of it. Western instruments do employ devices called resonators, which are merely shaped boxes designed to increase the amplitude of the instruments. This is why, for instance, a cello is not merely a piece of wood with strings. The hollowed body of the cello is its resonator. Since electronic instruments are amplified artificially, they do not require resonator boxes, which is why an electric guitar *is* merely a piece of wood, or even plastic.

An important element of resonance that is lacking in music healers' theories is the concept of periodicity; that is, for an object to have a resonant frequency, a pitch at which it vibrates, it must be (1) elastic, (2) prone to return to its original position and shape, and (3) when this elastic body is in motion it must move in a regular fashion at a concise and unwavering rate. A string that vibrates at 200 Hz vibrates precisely 200 times a second, not 190 one moment and 210 the next. When an object does not fulfill any one of these three criteria, it cannot resonate.

Peter Guy Manners reveals his lack of understanding of resonance in "Electrobiodynamics," writing,

> All matter is understood to have a rate of vibration which is peculiar to itself, notwithstanding that it may be imperceptible to normal human faculties or to detection by scientific instrumentation. To have a rate for vibration is to have rhythmical pattern of recurring periods wherein the

energy of the vibration changes from one value to another. In such a situation the frequency of a system is said to oscillate or exhibit rhythmic variations between certain maximum values. All matter, all freely vibrating systems then are conceived as having their own natural frequencies or periods of free oscillation. This constitutes a system's native vibration in an unobstructed state, i.e., without the influence of an outside compelling vibratory force. Resonance is said to occur when the respective periods of free oscillation of two or more different systems both having the same naturally occurring frequency are joined together in phase, resonance occurs with the result that their maximum and minimum values are reached simultaneously. Both systems vibrate in unison. Under these conditions the resultant wavelength values created by the union of the two frequencies exceed that which either could produce independently. An illustration of this is found in the fact that a vibrating tuning fork of the same [frequency] will set into sympathetic vibration or resonance another tuning fork of the same frequency.

Resonance, necessarily, involves an exchange between systems, a kind of mutual "sensing." In most cases when two vibrating systems interact, one becomes dominant and the other moves to the frequency of the dominant one.[1]

It is interesting that Manners illustrates his mistaken notion of bodies forcing other bodies to *change* their frequency with two tuning forks that are the same frequency. It is true that a 440-Hz tuning fork can cause resonance in another 440-Hz tuning fork, but one can play a 440-Hz tuning fork next to a 490-Hz fork for eternity and never will the 490-Hz fork resonate. Manners is also confusing vibration with pitch. An object can only have a pitch if it vibrates periodically. He says all matter has a rate of vibration, but he says also that the rate is variable. What is the meaning of the word *rate* then? If an object can vibrate at different rates and does, it will not produce a periodic vibration, and hence, will remain silent. A violin can produce an infinite number of pitches, but this is only because one is changing the length of the string employed. When one plucks the G string without altering its length, one produces a G, and nothing else, ever, as long as the exact length and tension are maintained. A cube of jello will oscillate, but it will not produce a sound because it does not oscillate at a fixed rate of speed. When Manners says that all matter has a rate of vibration that is peculiar to itself, he unwittingly denies the very possibility of resonance, which relies on the concept of sameness. All matter does oscillate. Carbon atoms oscillate; oxygen atoms oscillate; molecules of carbon dioxide oscillate; complex proteins made up of carbon, oxygen, hydrogen, and nitrogen oscillate; one-celled, living organisms oscillate; and we oscillate. But all matter does not oscillate periodically. When the G string of the violin is plucked, all the atoms in the string are oscillating, but that is irrelevant to the acoustical phenomenon of sound. Only the periodic oscillation of the string is relevant to sound. Sound is not synonymous with vibration.

Manners's misunderstanding of acoustics is captured in his conviction that periodicity can be characterized as having a "rate of vibration wherein the energy of the vibration changes from one value to another." This statement defines *aperiodicity,* not periodicity. Aperiodic vibration is that in which the rate of vibration changes. When Manners states that frequencies are periods of free oscillation, he is reversing the meaning of the word *frequency.* Frequency is fixed oscillation. If the oscillation is free, there is no frequency. Manners's definition of resonance as dependent upon "phase" is wrong and his statement that the two resonating bodies somehow cooperate to produce greater energy is pure nonsense. No energy is created by resonance. There is not "mutual sensing." There is a simple, well-understood process whereby an original sound source affects another sound source through a medium (such as air) and, as in all similar physical processes, energy is dissipated through friction, not amplified by "mutual sensing." If resonance disobeyed the reality of entropy, then once one started a second tuning fork resonating to a first, there would be no end to the escalation of amplitude. You can try this experiment in your home without fear of ear damage due to increasing amplification. Sound dies away unless energy is introduced to renew it.

Contrary to Manners's belief, one vibrating body does not become dominant, forcing another to change its frequency. A tuning fork of one frequency cannot coerce a tuning fork of another frequency to change its frequency.

Entrainment

Where it is easy to ascertain the nature of Manners's errors (his many errors in the excerpt above consist basically of a simple reversal of reality), Jonathan Goldman uses an "as if" process for his theorizing. Simplistic schemes are preferred without proof only to become accepted dogma moments later. "Living things are like television sets, in that living things also oscillate."[2] Goldman uses this metaphor to explain that living things can transmit images and ideas through a method similar to the method by which a television set receives its images (before cable television). Never mind that to make his point Goldman should say that living things are like broadcasting stations; he should also know that televisions do not oscillate, they receive oscillating signals.

"Entrainment is also found throughout nature. Fireflies blinking on and off will entrain with each other,"[3] Goldman writes. Goldman wants to establish a universal principle of resonance, or "entrainment." Like Manners he is unwilling to accept the real criteria for resonance and chooses to hypothesize about a resonance embedded in all aspects of nature. Referring to synchronized fireflies, Goldman explains that, "These rhythms of life allow for entrainment,"[4] when in fact a field of fireflies at night serves only to illustrate the stochastic and random principles of nature. "Such entrainment also takes place when two people have a good conversation. Their brain waves will oscillate synchronously. Such entrainment is seen in the relationship between students and their professors. Psychotherapists and clients entrain with each other. So do preachers and their congregation. As a matter of fact, you're probably entraining with me now."[5]

I don't think so. Goldman's entrainment theory is fabricated with half-remembered stories that do not bear up to scrutiny. He cites synchronized fireflies, ignoring the chaotic reality outside his window. Perhaps Goldman is recalling references to an Asian species of firefly he heard about at a New Age conference, but his recollection is never clarified. Goldman has never seen a pasture filled with fireflies blinking in unison. He has never been in a room full of grandfather clocks, either, though he asserts that, "If you have a room full of pendulum type grandfather clocks and start these pendulums in motion at different times, they will all being [*sic*] swinging differently. However, if you walk out of this room and come back the next day, you will find that all the pendulums are swinging together at the same rate. This locking in step of rhythms is entrainment. This was discovered by Huyghens in 1665."⁶

Huyghens did not discover whatever Goldman is claiming. Huyghens, a mathematician, physicist, and astronomer, is credited with many accomplishments, but no theories on "entrainment." Regarding pendulums, he discovered the utility of using them in clocks. He did no experiments with rooms full of them. Half-remembered stories and wishful thinking are the hallmark of Goldman's science. Goldman claims that, "It has been found that the frequencies of pulse, breathing and blood circulation, as well as their combined activities, all function harmonically. That is, their rhythms are strictly coordinated in whole number ratios— two to one, three to two."⁷ Unfortunately, Goldman offers a menu of brain-wave frequencies that do not reduce to the whole-number ratios. He reports that the alpha-wave spectrum of the human brain is identical to the Schumann effect, noting that the Schumann effect is 7.83 cycles per second. He also reports that delta signals of the brain are "1.5 cycles per second."⁸ Likewise Goldman notes that the theta signal is 4 cps. Needless to say, there is no simple, whole-number ratio between his figures. If, as Goldman writes, the delta signal is 1.5 cps and the theta signal 4 cps, then how does he reconcile these numbers with the "Schumann Effect," heart beat and breath, in whole-number ratios? They cannot be reconciled because they are not in whole-number ratios, and so Goldman refutes his own theory.

Goldman assumes that heart rate and respiration are periodic. For Goldman's entrainment ideas to be applicable he is assuming that our heart beats as "periodically" as a simple monochord or violin string, and, more incredibly, that our breathing rate is also periodic. Our actual breathing rate is so variable as to be completely unusable in a comparison to frequency. A rate of 60 cps cannot mean an average of 60 cps, but must be a regular, clockwork, 60 cps.

Even more simplistic is Steven Halpern's belief that breath rate and heart beat can be locked into a unison rhythm with a snap of a finger. Demonstrating this belief in his 1988 Music and Health Conference lecture, Halpern snapped his fingers and said, "Any external rhythm will . . . grab hold of your heart beat and your breath rate, immediately and inexorably and therefore you are controlling someone else's heartbeat."[9]

Apparently Halpern has discovered a cure for an immense range of ailments. If he is correct, he deserves the Nobel Prize as well as the eternal gratitude of the millions of people who have been exercising daily in order to decrease their heart rate. However, just like Goldman's fireflies, Halpern's finger-snap control of heart beat and breath rate is utterly disproved by reality. If you set a metronome at 50 beats per minute, you will find it impossible to align your heartbeat with 50, 100, or 150 beats per minute. It is difficult enough to consciously align your nonautonomic processes with it. Halpern can no more control my "breath rate" than he can my opinions, as both are subject to my conscious control.

Goldman and Halpern share a simplistic and mechanistic view of the world in which complex phenomena are reducible to whole-number ratios and finger-snap control. The odd thing about their viewpoints is that they belie their apparent perspective with a contradictory claim to a holistic philosophy of health, hearing, and humanity. According to Goldman,

In order to understand the holistic model of music, it is necessary to move from a mechanistic viewpoint—one that views internal organs, for example, as separate, isolated objects, unrelated to each other and the body as a whole—and come to the realization that not only are our internal parts interrelated to each other, but also to the mind and the spirit. The body, mind, spirit holistic model is certainly not new, but with music it becomes self-evident. Music—and specific frequencies in particular-can affect the organs, bones, and tissues right down to the cellular level. Different sounds can affect different parts of the brain as well, stimulating a variety of responses from the release of endorphins to the synchronization of the left and right hemispheres. Music can induce different states of consciousness, enhance or alter specific emotional and mental responses, and overall, affect our entire being. What else is there which has such a powerful effect on all aspects of the holistic self?[10]

But, what is *less* holistic than thinking a C natural will cure some specific ailment, that the cause of illness is irrelevant so long as we can treat a symptom? Goldman seems to recognize the philosophical problems with a healing theory that is not holistic, but in his article, "Sonic Entrainment and the Brain," he not only enthuses about therapeutic treatments that divide the body into separate distinct entities, but goes even further, suggesting that specific mental conditions can be treated by specific frequencies keyed to specific brain-wave frequencies. Goldman says in the article that the frequency of the earth is 7.83 cycles per second, which is "identical to the alpha wave spectrum of the human brain." Drop, for the moment, any objections to Goldman's assumption of a specific earth/human frequency and instead ask what such a philosophy of universal conformity has to do with holistic health concepts. In addition, who does Goldman mean to complain about in regard to a "mechanistic viewpoint"? What could be more mechanistic than the above-mentioned philosophy? If Goldman means to attack the Western medical tradition he ought to choose an alternative less, not more, restrictive than the Western model.

Resonating Bodies

The pitch material of New Age music is no different than that of all other Western music. The music healer cannot claim that he uses any specific frequencies more than any other composer and is thus more holistic or therapeutic. "A" natural occurs as many times (and more) in Beethoven's Seventh Symphony as it does in Steven Halpern's *Spectrum Suite.* But New Age music healers like to portray their compositions as containing some magical elixir of life that Beethoven's Seventh does not. This requires the music healer to claim that the pitches used in his pieces are scientifically and—paradoxically—spiritually selected for therapeutic purposes. The pitches music healers select, they claim, will resonate with the listener's body. Halpern and friends assign specific pitches to specific body parts. But, as if this were not simplistic enough, they further reduce humanity to a single overall pitch, and then concurrently expand the individual in such a way as to assign specific pitches for every organ and even brain function. Thus, they say, their music uniquely captures the human organism, hopeful, perhaps, that all of this talk will hide the fact that their music contains frequencies no different in quantity or quality than the latest Madonna pop single.

There is a more important flaw in their argument: that the human organism has an identifiable frequency; in fact, it does not. The human body does not resonate at any frequency. For an object to resonate it must vibrate periodically. "By periodic motion," explains Helmholtz, "we mean one which constantly returns to the same condition after exactly equal intervals of time."[11] That qualifier, "exactly," is essential to the understanding of frequency. Saying that humans breathe x number of times a minute does not establish a vibratory rate of breath because the breaths do not come at exact intervals. Furthermore, in addition to the prerequisite of periodicity there is the necessity of acoustical "elasticity," which includes a hypothetical state of rest. If you could arrange to stretch a human being's body between two points and cause him to undulate periodically (without killing him) it is conceivable that he could resonate. Or, if you could blow through one or the other end of his digestive/excretory system, he might produce a sound, but the frequencies produced in either operation would differ with each individual based on his height, weight, length of intestine, and so on.

As no one has successfully brought about either circumstance, it is curious that so many New Age music healers seem to know the precise frequency of the human body. There are, of course, certain human processes that produce sound. The vocal cords do, but the music healer prefers to ignore this quotidian reality. Also, brain waves constitute electrical, periodical phenomena; but as these frequencies are known throughout the medical community, and as they vary depending upon the individual and the type of brain function, these electrical (not sonic) frequencies are of no use in assaying a human resonance. (It should be noted that the electrical phenomena of the brain are too weak to escape the confines of the skull, so the various brain-wave measurement devices of such "tools" as the Betar, which do not use electrodes actually touching the scalp, cannot measure brain wave activity.)

These facts have not deterred New Age music healers from claiming a specific human frequency. Steven Halpern writes, "I am designing background music environments attuned to the human harmonic," and then informs his reader that it is no "mere 'coincidence' that the fundamental harmonic of our planet is identical to the fundamental harmonic of a tuned human body," which he identifies as "approximately 7.8 cycles per second," and two pages later as "about 7.5 cycles per second," and shortly thereafter as low as 6.8 cycles per second.[12] (The difference between 7.5 and 7.8 cycles per second is approximately a semitone; between 6.8 and 7.8 a whole tone—no minor difference in Halpern's figures.) Seven cycles per second, according to Halpern, is the resonant state of the meditating human body, making the meditator a full tone out of tune with the normal human. But in *Sound Health*, Halpern and Savary report that the resonant state of the meditating human body is 8 cycles per second. Also, whereas Halpern originally calculated the earth's frequency from the ionosphere-earth "Schumann effect," in *Sound Health,* Halpern and Savary redefine the Schumann resonance as calculated by "the speed of electro-magnetic radiation divided by the circumference of the Earth. The nervous systems of all life forms are attuned to this fundamental frequency."[13]

Let us attempt to clarify this hodge-podge of differing figures. Halpern states that the human being has a specific frequency. However, he gives several different frequencies as being the only frequency. One might argue that they are all within 2 cycles per second of each other. But due to the extremely low frequency he is discussing, the differences amount to a major second or more. Apparently Halpern is unaware of this difference in pitch. As for the pitch of the earth, Halpern gives different figures as well, and calculates them from completely different phenomenon, which, of course, explains why they are so different. Why the most obvious criteria for the earth's vibration are not used by music healers (specifically its periods of rotation, revolution, or wobble) is inexplicable. In regard to the human frequency, Halpern and his brethren justify a selection of 7.83 cps because, they say, it reflects the human brain in a meditative state. It does not. The 7.83 cps figure is merely one of an infinite number of meditative brain-wave frequencies that can be selected from a range of frequencies that centers around the borderline of the alpha (8 to 13 cycles per second) and the theta (4 to 8 cycles per second) electroencephalogram (EEG) brain-wave patterns. If we accept, for the sake of argument, that the range of this borderline, about 5 cycles per second, which is electronic and not sonic, is still a viable range for the frequency of a human being, we are talking about an interval of more than an octave from which we may choose the human frequency. In other words, any pitch whatsoever can be chosen and defended using the low alpha or high theta wave frequency as the criterion for *the* human frequency. Besides the fact that any pitch within this low octave could be selected as the human frequency, there is no reason for choosing this particular brain-wave frequency or, for that matter, any brain-wave frequency; but the choice of 7.83 as representing *the* alpha (or theta) brain wave is dishonest.

If, as Halpern and Savary claim, all life shares the same fundamental "Schumann" frequency, then why do they note, "Different parts of our bodies resonate at different frequencies. Each human organ may have its own keynote frequency." Halpern and Savary are badly misinformed about sound. "We know," they mistakenly assert, "that crystals, violins, bodily organs—in fact, all physical matter—produce detectable 'tones.' The phenomenon of resonance, or sympathetic vibration, is not contingent on volume, but on pitch."[14] If they had read their Helmholtz they would know that resonance *is* contingent on amplitude (force), which they lazily cite as volume, *and* frequency, not pitch. (Pitch is not as definite as frequency—440 cps and 450 cps are both the "pitch" A, but a 440 cps object will not resonate to a 450 cps source.) Without enough amplitude a source cannot transmit its vibratory rate through the medium to the resonant body. For example, a 440 cps tuning fork will not cause another 440 cps tuning fork to resonate if its amplitude is too low or the forks' distance from each other is sufficient to reduce the apparent amplitude below a prerequisite threshold.

Goldman writes,

> It is interesting to note, that the Earth's ionosphere, the electromagnetic field around the earth has been measured. This is called the Shumann [sic] Effect, and it appears that this frequency of the Earth is somewhere around 7.83 cycles per second. This is identical to the alpha wave spectrum of the human brain. It has been speculated that when we meditate, our brain waves lock in and entrain with the energies of the earth.
>
> Itzhak Bentov speculated that perhaps when a person was vibrating at these frequencies during meditation, they would entrain with the Earth and lock in resonance with it.[15]

Such a person will not resonate if, according to Halpern, who also cites Bentov, he is a major second out of tune with the earth. Goldman gives the meditating human body the frequency of 7.83 cps, but he cites no evidence for this presumption. Halpern gives the figure of 7.0 cps for the meditative frequency and 7.83 as the Earth's frequency. These are not resonant frequencies.

Sharing the view of a specific Earth resonance is Don Campbell. He sees a lack of proper resonance as causing cancer. "The brain becomes entrained to sounds after a short period of time and literally does not hear them. Yet the body is always aware of the sound. We are made aware of the dangers of inaudible low-frequency drones from power lines above our homes by the alarming upsurge of cancer in those who live nearby. These rhythms are so out of harmony with the earth's drone of 7.8 vibrations per second that people between this sound and the earth incur disease."[16]

Perhaps the most inept characterization of the human frequency is that of William David in *The Harmonics of Sound, Color and Vibration*. He writes, "The pitch of your speaking voice is your natural sound frequency."[17] By this does he mean the pitch of your speaking voice in the morning, the evening, when excited, when calm, when speaking to a friend, to a stranger? Does he not know that many languages (such as Thai) use differing frequencies to differentiate between different sounds? For example, in Thai, the sentence "Mai mai mai mai" means "New wood burns, doesn't it?" The first "mai" is spoken in the high register, the second in the low register, the third begins at mid-range and descends to a lower register, the fourth begins in a lower register and ascends. Not included in the sentence is the common Thai mid-range syllable. The Thai language requires these five different inflections; does David believe that Thai people have a minimum of five frequencies? Americans use many different frequencies, too, but these are not used to differentiate between words, though the use of frequency alteration is necessary for the understanding of spoken English. For instance, the sentence "New wood burns," as a declarative remark generally ends with the word "burns" lower in frequency than "new wood." However, in the question, "New wood burns?" the word "burns" is higher in frequency. There is no "pitch" to the human voice, so deriving a "natural sound frequency" from such a fiction is, of course, impossible.

The concept of a single healthy human pitch is determined in a manner wholly consistent with behaviorism, rather than the spirit of holism. In the behavioral model there exist specific desired responses that are positively rewarded while noncompliant responses may be negatively reinforced or ignored. The purpose of behaviorism is to enforce a pre-identified "appropriate" response. Health is defined as adherence to a predefined model of correctness. The holistic model, on the other hand, defines health as a state of growth appropriate for the individual, and eschews the concept of a predefined, universal, correct model of behavior. Whereas the behaviorist has as his goal the alteration of what is considered maladaptive responses, the holistic therapist views the condition in question as an opportunity to explore this aspect of the personality in order to further one's potential in life. Alteration is not the goal of holistic therapy; self-awareness and growth is. Becoming "normal," or the same as others, is not the goal of holistic therapy; becoming an individual is. In the supposed holistic field of New Age music healing, nearly all of the practitioners prescribe a specific frequency as necessary for right behavior, right thought, and a healthy body. If one does not vibrate at 7.83 cps, then one is out of tune and must be fixed. How less holistic can music healing be than for the healer to decide that one frequency out of infinite possibilities is the only acceptable, and healthy, one at which to oscillate?

"Movable" healing tones have proven to be too complicated a procedure for our Western New Age music healers. Most prefer a simple one-to-one relationship with no transposition. Since the tone C is red (though C can be any of various different frequencies) then, those healers suggest, C must cure one specific group of symptoms. Kay Gardner reports that a treatment of five minutes at 40 Hz, five minutes at 60 Hz, five minutes at 80 Hz, and five minutes at 40 Hz again will relieve back, shoulder, and neck pain. Gardner claims that Bechterer's disease should be treated with 44, 58, and 88 Hz. For menstrual pain, asthma, and cystic fibrosis, Gardner prescribes a "50 Hz root, fifth, octave, root sequence."[18] In the program notes to her *Garden of Ecstacy* tape Gardner reveals that through "years of research on music as a healing force, including how particular tones and key centers affect the human organism," she had determined that the pitch F♯ "touches the mid-chest area of the body where the thymus, the 'brain' of the immune system is located." Having established this to her satisfaction, she composed "Viriditas" to "fight against AIDS."[19]

In fact, Gardner wants her beliefs that specific illnesses can be cured by specific frequencies taught in colleges, especially in music education and music therapy programs. "Composition students could learn the healing and therapeutic elements of music and could incorporate such knowledge into their compositions. Theory classes could concentrate more on research in the effects of the old modal melodies in the healing process, and how particular intervals stimulate certain emotions."[20]

Halpern suggests, in *Tuning the Human Instrument,* "If someone is deficient in the functioning of a liver, for instance, instead of just giving them vitamin A, one might receive a portion of sound vibrations—vitamin A-sharp. Interestingly, these sound stimuli can be transduced directly into the skin, so that there is actually *no* sound that is heard, by patient or technician."[21]

While Halpern's theorizing on a pitch to cure liver ailments may seem laughable, his themes are not without supporters in the field of music therapy. Halpern's books, his questionable research, his lectures are taken quite seriously and soberly by a growing number of professionals. Even music therapists who are trained in the scientific method, proper research, music theory, and acoustics can be hoodwinked by the smoke and mirrors of scientific-sounding treatises. Music therapists are increasingly embracing the dubious theories of New Age music healers. Mathematical equations, official-looking abbreviations ("ELFs," "CPS," and the like), and neologisms crowd the pages of sundry theories of music healing, disguising their lack of real scientific foundation.

Out of the Body

One New Ager who has flooded the market with confusing jargon and confused acoustical healing principles is Robert Monroe, whose birth as a New Age guru occurred in the 1950s, when he began having out-of-body experiences, which he labeled acronymically OOBEs. In his first book, *Journeys Out of the Body*, Monroe describes his experience as a noncorporeal traveler in several worlds. Humans, he explains, can leave their bodies behind during sleep and fly to various locations of earth, not in their dreams or imagination, but in reality. Monroe tells us that he could be asleep in his home while simultaneously in another room hundreds of miles away, sometimes visible, sometimes invisible, sometimes observing but sometimes actively participating in events. Monroe writes that his OOBEs were so commonplace that when his eldest daughter went to college, before she and her roommate would undress for bed she would say, "Daddy, if you're here, I think you better go now. We want to get undressed for bed."[22] Much of Monroe's OOBE experiences revolve around sex and titillating situations. The obvious opportunity for Monroe to spy upon people unawares presented a moral dilemma for him. In his book, Monroe struggles for several chapters with the guilt he feels about his sexual desires. In the late 1950s he realized that his sexual restraint was imposed on him by an unenlightened society. Subsequently, he was freed to have sexual relationships with those he met during his OOBEs. Monroe reports that an orgasm can be reached (in an alternate world he labels "location two") by the employment of a sexually charged special "handshake." Other times more prosaic means are used. In March 1961, Monroe reports, a friend of his wife visited his home.

> I decided to sleep in the study, rather than in the bedroom with my wife, as I felt that I could induce the vibrations and didn't want possibly to disturb her sleep. . . . After many preliminaries, the vibrations came in strong and accelerated to a frequency beyond perception as individual

pulsations. I lifted out of the physical easily, and . . . went on up, through the ceiling and floor above. . . . The room was dark, and I was sure I was in the children's bedroom, but could see no one. I was about to try to go somewhere else when I became aware of a woman in the room not too far from me. . . . She was a woman of considerable sexual experience. This latter sense brought forth my sex drive, and I was attracted to her. As I approached, she said she would "rather not," because she was very tired. I moved back respecting her wishes. . . . Then I noticed a second woman . . . older than the first, in her 40's but also a woman of wide sexual experience. The second woman moved forward and offered to "be" with me. . . . I needed no further invitation . . . and we moved together quickly. There was the giddy electrical-type shock, and then we separated. Feeling this was enough for one night, I turned and dived through the floor and soon was re-entering the physical. . . . I smoked a cigarette and then lay down and slept for the rest of the night.[23]

The morning after his adulterous OOBE tryst, Monroe encouraged his wife to question their overnight guest, whom he calls "J.F."

I asked my wife to go up and ask J.F. if she was sexually "tired." She asked me what I meant and I explained. Then, of course, she wanted to know why, and said that she couldn't ask J.F. such a question. I said I was sure she could find out, that it was important. Finally, she agreed and went upstairs to awaken J.F. I waited for a long time and finally my wife came back downstairs alone. She looked at me intently.

"How did you know?" Thank goodness she did not ask it suspiciously. . . . A short time later J.F. came down for breakfast. My wife . . . had not told her anything of my interest in her condition. I caught her staring at me intently again and again, as if she were trying to remember something about me but couldn't. I gave no indication that I noticed this sudden interest. This was fairly good identification.[24]

In the above excerpt Monroe reveals his method for establishing the veracity of his noncorporeal visitations. He remarks that J. F. was staring at him intently "again and again," and that this, in his opinion, was "fairly good" proof that his trip upstairs through the ceiling was no mere wet dream.

Lest I give the wrong impression, Monroe's OOBEs were not undertaken solely for sexual gratification, though sexual episodes seem to predominate his recollections. Monroe also visited astral monks and had a conversation with his deceased father; both of these visitations were to another "location." The motivating factor behind Monroe's OOBEs is apparently his contact with an extraterrestrial plenipotentiary who was looking for a suitable representative from earth for an intergalactic United Nations. Once earth is able to join the "intergalactic society" then "misdirected fantasies and conjecture" will be "gone immediately." The earth has not been invited to join this union because the extraterrestrials have been unable to successfully contact earthlings due to a "virtually unbearable psi noise." This psi noise is the result of human irrationality, "uncontrolled and non-objective." Nevertheless, one plucky alien was brave enough to "establish physical contact . . . while the others wait patiently in a shelter on the planet's barren and brittle satellite." (By this Monroe means that the rest of the aliens are hiding out on the moon.) Almost all of those the alien contacts "lose their ability to reason, and are isolated as sufferers of some disease. Any lasting psi communication pattern is usually labeled as unreality or dream."[25] Monroe reports that our potential benefactors in the intergalactic society are hampered by the intellectual leaders of the earth, and that their only success has been with

> individuals without inhibitory "scientific" training. With little to unlearn and no prestige loss to be suffered, productive exchange of rational thought has been accomplished in several of these relatively uneducated inhabitants. . . . The work still continues. High-level psi force radiation equipment is being employed in the hope of a breakthrough to the society members during their waking, active state. Any individuals who possess some degree of intellect coupled with objective curiosity are being taught, sometimes painfully, the basics of psi force techniques.[26]

In 1971 when Monroe wrote of psi force education, New Age music healing was at a nadir, and the people of the United States were more preoccupied with the politics of Vietnam and social changes here and abroad. Most New Age subjects took a back seat to the more earthly concerns of the late sixties and early seventies. A book like *Journeys Out of the Body* was largely irrelevant to the philosophy of those volatile times, but proved a prescient foreshadowing of current New age thinking. Laboring in relative obscurity, Monroe realized the vision of the psi force school, founding the Monroe Institute and creating its curriculum. The program for psi force enlightenment, the Gateway Program, was infused with his extraterrestrial philosophy and a naive concept of acoustics. Monroe's OOBEs became the linchpin of the "research," which was conducted on entrainment of the brain to specific frequencies. Monroe declared that his OOBEs could be triggered by sound, and that through resonance one could entrain the brain. He called his discovery a "frequency following response," and reportedly patented the effect in 1975.

In *Journeys Out of the Body* there are hints of what is yet to come. In order to experience an OOBE, Monroe asserts, one must mentally direct vibrations into a ring about the body, sweeping the rings rhythmically "from head to toes and then back again." The frequencies of these mental vibrations are rough at first, he says, and there will be

> a desire to "smooth" them out. This is accomplished by "pulsing" them mentally to increase their frequency. Their original vibratory rate seems to be on the order of some 27 cps (this is the rate of the vibration itself, not the head to toe frequency). . . . The faster vibration effect is the form that permits disassociation from the physical. Once you have set the momentum of the speed up, the acceleration seems to take place automatically. Eventually, you may sense the vibrations only as they begin. They will increase their frequency—like a motor starting up—until the frequency is so high that you are unable to perceive it. . . . Another word of warning is in order here, beyond this point I believe you cannot turn back.[27]

And Monroe did not turn back. Perhaps he recognized that his "dis-association" process lacked the jargon and pseudoscientific gibberish necessary to elevate it to a level of acceptance. His institute and Gateway Program retain the goal of his OOBE writing, but dramatically alter the supposed acoustical process necessary for entering an OOBE. The original 27 cps start-up frequency followed by a revving up beyond audible sound lacked credibility and offered no commercial advantage to Monroe the businessman. In 1971, the noncorporeal traveler was instructed by Monroe to duplicate his OOBEs, which numbered in the thousands, by raising his own body frequency in an unaided way through mental will. In 1971, Monroe required no machines for those who wished to follow in his footsteps, and the only prerequisite for inducing OOBEs was reading the sixteenth and seventeenth chapters of his book.

But a decade later Monroe's philosophy and acoustical requirements were radically different. In order to undergo an OOBE, pocket change for a paperback book would no longer do. One needed to attend the Monroe Institute and experience the "Hemi-Synch" phenomenon, possible only through this special training program.

Participants in Monroe's Gateway Program use Hemi-Synch to "establish methods of contact with other energy forms." Not only does the participant establish contact, but he learns to converse with these extraterrestrial forms, to "speak and report using normal language . . . to conduct and maintain rational dialogue . . . to retain full conscious awareness and memory of the communication."[28] It will not do to merely phone E.T.; you want to be able to talk about your conversation. The Gateway Voyage, a six-day trip to the Monroe Institute, costs only $1,195. The graduate study trip, to the same locale, costs another $1,195. There are further seminars that cost $1,495 each, including "marketing materials." This is a unique and lucrative travel bureau venture for Monroe. He doesn't even need to share his profits with an airline.

The price is trivial compared to the effects that Monroe believes he and his followers are having upon the universe. In *Journeys Out of the*

Body Monroe suggests that during the out-of-body experience a person can effect world-shaking changes with ease.

> Before dismissing this as an absurdity, consider that I was able to affect another living human being physically in the "pinching" episode. If one can do this, so can others. Nothing more than a pinch at the right time in the right place in the physical body of another human being can change the world. It takes little imagination to visualize a pinched cerebral artery in the brain as the cause of the stroke in a world leader. . . . All that is needed is the ability and the intent. . . . Further, a person operating in the Second Body [OOBE] can affect other human beings mentally.[29]

Entraining the Brain

The Monroe Institute brochure claims:

> Certain sound patterns create a Frequency Following Response (FFR) in the electrical activity of the brain. These blended and sequenced sound patterns can gently lead the brain into various states, such as deep relaxation or sleep. A generic patent in this field was issued to Robert Monroe in 1975. Drawing upon this discovery and the work of others, Mr. Monroe employed a system of "binaural beats" by feeding a separate signal into each ear. By sending separate sound pulses to each ear with stereo headphones, the two hemispheres of the brain act *in unison* to "hear" a third signal—the difference between the two sound pulses. This third signal is not an actual sound, but an electrical signal that can only be created *by both brain hemispheres acting and working together, simultaneously.*
>
> The unique coherent brain state that results is known as hemispheric synchronization, or "Hemi-Synch." The audio stimulus which creates this state is not overpowering. It is noninvasive and can easily be disregarded either objectively or subjectively.[30]

This, in a nutshell, is Monroe's Hemi-Synch concept. It is the basis of all the work of the Monroe Institute and the Gateway Program. Monroe's hypothesis is simple. One, brain waves can be modified by the introduction of a subjective tone heard only in the brain, not part of the physical process of audition taking place in the ears; two, the subjective tone is created by playing pitches of two slightly differing frequencies, thus causing the phenomenon of beats, which Monroe considers synonymous to these subjective tones; and three, these beats are created by the technique of transmitting the two frequencies separately, one to the left ear and one to the right ear, at subsonic levels through headphones.

Not one of these three elements holds water. Regarding the first, sonic frequencies are not translated to brain-wave frequency on a one-to-one or harmonic basis—440 cps is not translated to 440 cps in brain wave frequency, or any particular ratios thereof.[31] If one introduces a tone of 440 cps in one ear and a tone of 445 cps in the other, the brain will not identify this 5 cps difference by comparing brain waves differing by 5 cps. The last place that the perceived sound of 440 cps is registered as physically real is in the inner ear prior to its translation into electrical impulses.

Monroe is also confused about the derivation of subjective tones. There is an argument among physiologists who study the audition of sound about the location of subjective tones. The argument has nothing to do with the brain, however, but rather with the inner ear. Subjective tones are called subjective because they do not exist outside the ear, but are produced as a result of the difference, in audition, of two simultaneous frequencies upon the inner ear itself. Helmholtz explains that the force of the combinational tone is generated in the ear itself; the auditory ossicles and drumskin vibrating sufficiently generate the combination tones. The vibrations that result do not exist in the external medium (air), but do exist, objectively, in the ear.[32] The question of subjectivity has nothing to do with the brain. It has to do with the interaction of frequencies within the ear itself in which are generated tones for which there is no external sound source. For instance, the simultaneous sonority of two pitches with the frequencies of 100 cps and 300 cps respectively, will produce the subjective difference tone of 200 cps. (There is also a subjective-summation tone of 400 cps, but neither Monroe nor any other music healers discusses the phenomenon of summation tones.) In this example, the difference tone produced is an octave above the 100 cps tone and a perfect fifth below the 300 cps tone. Because the ear cannot discriminate between the two objective tones it receives coming from an outside source and the subjective tone(s) created within it, the brain remains unaware of the origin of the 200 cps tone. In effect, Monroe has gotten the phenomenon completely backwards by assuming that the brain, rather than the ear, is producing the subjective tone.[33]

As if it were not enough to sink Monroe's Hemi-Synch that his understanding of the physiological aspects of subjective tones upon which he bases his methods contradicts reality, Monroe is also unaware of the difference between subjective tones and "beats." Subjective tones are not beats, though they are related on a mathematical level. For instance, two cellists playing the pitch A, but at slightly differing frequencies, will cause beats. If one cellist's A is 220 cps and the other cellist's A is 225 cps, there will be a resultant 5-beats-per-second wobble in the combination of their sounds. This beat phenomenon is amplitude modulation, the result of the two wave fronts of the slightly differing frequencies interfering with each other. When the crest of one wave coincides with the trough of the other, a form of sound cancellation occurs. Likewise, when crests coincide, there is an intensification of sound. In music worldwide, beats of up to 5 per second are not heard as annoying, but above 5 beats per second, the sound is disagreeable to human ears, increasing in unpleasantness as the beats increase. If we hear two instruments playing the same pitch at frequencies differing by 15 cps we complain that they are out of tune. Above 30 beats per second, the wobble is too fast for human ears to distinguish, and the beat phenomenon ends. At this point, the beats themselves may be construed by the inner ear as a new and subjective pitch. The beat phenomenon under 30 cps is amplitude modulation. But above 30 cps the regular undulations of amplitude are so fast as to escape detection as amplitude modulation, and if detectable at all, enter the realm of frequency. Monroe's binaural beats are *not* above 30 cps; therefore, they do not create a subjective tone, and, unlike subjective tones, they are objectively real since they are transmitted through the air just as are the frequencies that caused them. Using a machine to register these beats is possible because these beats are an objective phenomenon. Beats are not frequency (nor are they tones, nor are they subjective tones). They are changes in loudness, and are a physical phenomenon that alters the transmission of sound in the air. Subjective tones have no effect upon the transmission of sound, nor upon the air. When Monroe equates beats with subjective tones he is confusing amplitude with frequency, and objective with subjective.

Monroe's technique for the creation of his misnamed subjective tones makes it impossible for them to occur. Subjective tones are created in the ear. As previously noted, they are the result of the interaction of separate frequencies in the ear. If the frequencies are separated, as Monroe requires, one going into the left ear, the other going into the right ear, there can be no interaction (the ears do not communicate with each other, they transmit to the brain). Recall the two frequencies of 100 cps and 300 cps. In the inner ear they combine (hence Helmholtz's label "combinational tones") to create the 200-cps subjective tone. Monroe's apparatus prohibits any interaction, and thus precludes the formation of the subjective tones. Likewise, his apparatus forbids the formation of beats. Beats are caused by the interaction of slightly differing frequencies in the air, causing the resultant wobble effect. However, if one sends a 220-cps signal to the left ear through a headphone and a 225-cps signal to the right ear, the waves cannot interfere with each other, so there can be no beat phenomenon, as Monroe is claiming. In either case, whichever he really means, beats or subjective tones, Monroe's method of producing them through headphones is the one sure method to prevent them from occurring.

Furthermore, as Monroe prescribes inaudible (subsonic) tones for the creation of his Hemi-Synch effect, as these inaudible tones do not have any physical effect upon the ear, and as we cannot hear them, *they* cannot cause beats nor subjective tones. They are inaudible, and as such are not detectable by our brains as auditory phenomena.[34]

Despite the myriad flaws in his Hemi-Synch procedure, Monroe cites "medically documented spontaneous remission of incurable illness" as a result of his methods.[35] That spontaneous remission of "incurable" illness occurs, I do not argue. That Hemi-Synch can cure "incurable" illness I find baseless and note that Monroe does not proffer evidence in support of this implication.

Monroe's backwards version of acoustics has found widespread acceptance in the New Age music-healing community, spawning music-healing theories in which Monroe's errors become the building blocks of subsequent theories. Jonathan Goldman is but one music healer who blindly, or should we say deafly, follows Monroe's lead.

> In order for this patented process, which Monroe called "Hemi-Sync" [*sic*] to work, it appeared that it was necessary for those hearing the two sound sources to wear headphones. Later work with the frequency following response however, indicated that entrainment of the brain would still occur with external sound sources, such as stereo speakers, for example, if they were given enough separation in the room. While the effects were not quite as rapid or as powerful as with headphones, entrainment still took place.[36]

If Goldman had researched the real experiments of acousticians, or even just read the appropriate chapter from any elementary acoustics book, he would have realized that the further the separation of the speakers, the *less* the possibility of combination tones or beats. Goldman is actually saying that hemispheric synchronization is accomplished by eliminating beats and subjective tones, which is, amusingly, in agreement with Monroe's practice. Goldman's problem lies in accepting Monroe's acoustical expertise as equivalent to his marketing expertise. Helmholtz's book *On the Sensations of Tone* did not make Helmholtz a wealthy man, but his verifiable experiments with beats and subjective tones did make him an expert on acoustics.

Music healers attempt to "cure" left brain dominance through Monroe's Hemi-Synch process. Implicit in this simplistic philosophy is the belief that thought processes should not be dominated by the left hemisphere of the brain. Peter Guy Manners, of Cymatics fame, has "researched" Hemi-Synch at Bretforton Hall Clinic under the auspices of "Bretforton Naturopathic Scientific Research." Speaking of the brain, Manners writes, "Most of the time, we think only with our 'left brain.' When we use our 'right brain,' it is primarily to support the thought and action of the left. Otherwise, we do our best to ignore it."[37]

Manners attempts a scientific explanation of the "frequency following response."

> Certain sound patterns create a Frequency Following Response (FFR) in the electrical activity of the brain. Those sound patterns can then lead the brain into various states, such as deep relaxation or sleep, a system of "binaural beats," feeding a separate signal into each ear. By sending separate sound pulses to each ear with stereo headphones, the two hemispheres of the brain act in unison to "hear" a third signal—the difference between the two sound impulses. This third signal is not an actual sound, but an electrical signal that can only be created by both brain hemispheres acting and working together simultaneously.[38]

This is only parroting Monroe's inept theories, but then Manners learned his acoustics from Hans Holt, not from Helmholtz.

Steven Halpern made a suggestion that, if it were true (and it is as true as Monroe's Hemi-Synch), would provide a substantial savings over the investment necessary to have your hemispheres balanced by Monroe. Of a Tibetan bowl he remarked, "As you spin it around it makes this very nice sound. Now, guaranteed, if you spend a moment or two with this it will balance the hemispheres of your brain."[39] There, Halpern just saved you a thousand dollars.

You could turn around and spend those thousand dollars you just saved on products from Dick Sutphen's Sutphen Corporation. Dick Sutphen, a New Age mass market sales guru, sells entrainment tapes, as well as subliminal tapes and straight lectures about his reincarnation/past-life philosophy. Sutphen advertises *Awakened Dreaming* as a "unique new tape [that] incorporates the scientific technology of cycles-per-second brain activity and frequency follow response. This is synthesized into an unusual sound that will alter your consciousness and open the door to your unconscious mind."[40] This is a simplistic avulsion of Monroe's Hemi-Synch. Sutphen gives no credit to Monroe, but it is obvious through his use of Monroe's jargon ("FFR") where Sutphen has gained his inspiration.

"The incredible Beta-to-Theta tape" is described in another advertisement.

Thousands of seminar participants and buyers have reported phenomenal results with Beta-to-Theta Sound Technique. There are four brain levels: Beta, Alpha, Theta and Delta. When you're wide awake you are in Beta. When you go into hypnosis or meditation you go into Alpha or Theta. The levels of the mind can be monitored at various cycles-per-second of activity. The way this tape works is as follows: cycles-per-second are converted into clicks-per-minute, and the tape begins with the rapid clicking sound of mid-Beta mental activity. As the sound is slowed down over a five-minute period, your mind synchronizes or locks onto the sound and slows down with it. When you relax and focus your full attention upon the sound you are effortlessly lulled into an altered state of consciousness. The sound stabilizes at the top of Theta (a deep meditative state) and continues to click at the speed for 25 more minutes. At this level, suggestion is accepted approximately 100 times as effectively as in a waking state.[41]

A DM-20 pocket digital metronome can click or beat at .5 cycles per second up to 16.66 cycles per seconds, and can be sped up or slowed down imperceptibly, but I cannot imagine a sane person actually subjecting himself to this for more than a couple of minutes. Sutphen's method for brain entrainment is no more absurd than Monroe's, only Sutphen has stripped more of the disguising jargon from the concept. Monroe wants to create a 4-cps frequency in the brain and claims he will do this by playing, for instance, a 7-cps frequency in the left ear and an 11-cps frequency in the right. This, he says, will create a subjective tone of 4 cps. Sutphen cuts out the middleman and simply plays a tape consisting of a 4-cps sound. In both cases the sonic cps will supposedly coerce the equivalent brain wave frequency and thus engender a synchronized brain, or meditative brain, or whatever particular state the New Age music healer wants to induce.

When the entraining sound is meant to correspond on a one-to-one basis with the brain-wave frequency the sound is inaudible, and hence cannot be transmitted to the brain from the ear. Sutphen claims to change cycles per second to clicks per minute. Sutphen is claiming that a frequency of 4 cps is heard by the ear if one plays four "clicks" in a second. You, of course, can do this by tapping your finger four times a second on wood, but you are not creating a frequency of 4 cps, you are creating a rhythm, or pulse. The four taps per second will not create a correspondent sonic wave form of 4 cps. Each tap (assuming you are not tapping a resonant object or an object with a pitch) engenders a single concussive wave front, not a periodic vibration. Thus, where Monroe confuses frequency with amplitude, Sutphen has confused frequency with rhythm. One might ask, at this point, why entrainment advocates do not simply place electrodes in the scalp and transmit electronic pulses with the frequencies they wish to entrain. The answer is: they would be arrested, because in the United States one needs a medical degree to run electricity through people's brains.

If you have managed to hold on to the money you saved by not going to Monroe's Gateway Program, and Sutphen's products did not interest you either, perhaps Robert Anton Wilson could interest you in some affordable sound-therapy devices.

Robert Anton Wilson, an author of fiction (the Illuminatus trilogy) and speculative paranormal literature has reviewed several sound-therapy machines. One of the machines Wilson experimented with was the "Pulstar," a machine that its inventor, Michael Hercules, claimed would synchronize the two hemispheres of the brain. The Pulstar merely plays low frequencies (from 4 to 30 cps as reported by Wilson). At 30 cps Wilson got a feeling "as if I had taken cocaine." This experience in "high beta" was followed by "moving back to alpha (8 to 13 Hz)," which Wilson found "especially soothing and relaxing." During his use of the Pulstar, Wilson claims to have experienced an out-of-body experience, as well as brain death.

> The range from 8 to 4 hz, called theta, proved . . . delightful to explore.
> . . . At 4 hz I had a classic "Out-of-Body-Experience," and . . . moved out of the lab, over the Rockies, up above the North Pole, swooped over Iceland, found Ireland and explored the peninsula of Howth. The most exciting part of this trip came after I "returned" to the lab. Mike Hercules had made an e.e.g. during my O.O.B.E. and showed it to me. I had no beta, no alpha, no theta, no delta—no brainwaves at all. The e.e.g. looked like that of a dead man. A flat line, like the ones in 2001 when the monitors flash LIFE FUNCTIONS TERMINATED.
>
> Later I explored delta (below 4 hertz), where it seems hard to stay awake and one "dreams" even if one does not stay awake. But I remembered most vividly the O.O.B.E. and the brainwave reading of the e.e.g., which showed that I had no brainwaves at all in the "out-of-body" state. I've been having O.O.B.E.s since about 1963, and have never known quite what to think of them. Looking at my flat, "dead" brainwaves during the Pulstar O.O.B.E., I felt that I knew more and understood less. Whatever was visualizing that trip over the Pole to Ireland, my brain evidently was not involved.[42]

No argument there. After "512 hours in cyberspace," Wilson had his "brainwaves" measured by Anna Wise. According to Wilson, she concluded that his "right/left balance" approximated that of "Zen masters she had measured," but that he had "some irregularities more typical of artists than mystics." Furthermore, she also found that I have a lot of delta even when awake—typical of psychics, she said.[43]

I would remind Wilson that as Wise did not measure his brainwaves prior to his "cyberspace" experiments, we cannot know if this is an improvement or a deterioration of his brain-wave patterns. Wilson does not find it ironic that the inventors of the machines he reviews find Wilson to be a superman.

Wilson's favorite electromagnetic trainer, as he calls these machines, is the "Endo-Max" stimulant tape: "Some physicians report success in using it to cure cocaine abuse—the tape seemingly teaches the brain how to speed up naturally, without the cocaine any longer being 'felt' as necessary. More research, of course, is needed before we start celebrating this as a 'cure' for all cocaine abuse problems."[44]

Wilson, though, is no stickler for details and is willing to claim medical confirmation and scientifically verified experiments when neither exist. This is a science-fiction vision and a trite one at that, shared by numerous New Age music healers who find that human salvation may be just around the corner in the form of machines. Jonathan Goldman enthuses, "These are exciting times with many new discoveries going on. People using frequencies and rhythms for relaxation, stress reduction and treatments for all sorts of illness and diseases. There's the Somatron, the Betar, Cymatic Therapy, Flyborg Therapy, and much more! . . . The implications of this . . . are quite astounding and far reaching. It is a great responsibility. And one we should be aware of."[45]

Special machines have been designed to cash in on a gullible public's belief in quick-fix entrees to transcendental states. The Isis, developed by Jack Schwarz, uses light pulses delivered through goggles to "entrain beta, alpha, theta, and delta brain frequencies." The Neuropep uses tapes that control light and sound frequencies in tandem. The David uses light, sounds, and Ericksonian hypnotic inductions. The Synchro-Energizer employs a computer in its offering of brain entrainment frequencies of light and sound. The Mc-Squared uses light and music, rather than just simple tones.[46] "Computerized brain machines are up there, a few years ahead," opines Wilson. "You will just sit down and keyboard in the brainwaves that you want. Full Zen Master pattern. Einstein pattern. Beethoven pattern."[47]

The part of Wilson's statement that can never be true is the silly conceit that Beethoven's "pattern" or Einstein's "pattern" could be garnered from a machine. They are dead. As for the "Zen Master," we are confident that no Zen master would ever offer his brain wave pattern to anyone else through the medium of a machine. If Wilson were to ask the Zen master for his brainwave pattern, I suspect the master would say,

The best of paths is Eightfold; the best of truths the Four Sayings; the best of virtues passionlessness; the best of men he who has eyes to see. This is the path, there is no other that leads to the purifying of the mind. Go on this path! This will confuse Mara the tempter. If you go on this way, you will make an end of pain—the way preached by me, when I had understood the removal of the thorns in the flesh. *You yourself must make an effort.* The Tathagatas [Buddhas] are only preachers. The thoughtful who enter the way are freed from the bondage of Mara. All created things perish—he who knows and sees this is at peace though in a world of pain; this is the way to purity. All created things are grief and pain—he who knows and sees this is at peace though in a world of pain; this is the way that leads to purity. All forms are unreal—he who knows and sees this is at peace though in a world of pain; this is the way that leads to purity. He who does not rouse himself when it is time to rise, who, though young and strong, is full of sloth, whose will and thought are weak, that lazy and idle man never finds the way to wisdom.[48]

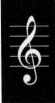

7. Research: Right Vocation

Psychotronic Experiments

When examining research by New Age music healers one is often stymied by a lack of data. "Research" is used as a word, but the data from this research is often nothing more than anecdote or wishful thinking. Nevertheless, music healers who use science in their research, and scientific jargon to support their views, open themselves up to proper scientific criticism. Very often, however, the "science" is merely a facade, a rationalization for irrational beliefs. Commenting on classical music, Steven Halpern transcribes an interview he had with Don West.

> We employed as our test selection a composition by Liszt that scored highest among listener agreement in the category of "Relaxing/Meditative/Soothing"—as defined by the Music Research Foundation, the agency set up by the U.S. Surgeon General's office to know about such things—the actual physical reaction was very much less than that which might have been expected. . . . In other words one might *think* that one was getting relaxed, but the scientific apparatus showed that music of this kind was not registered in the body; i.e., the electromagnetic energy field and the electrical conductivity of the skin were not altered into deep relaxational parameters.[1]

Halpern would have his reader believe that the "relaxational parameters" have been defined by a Relaxation Research Foundation set up by the U.S. Surgeon General's office "to know about such things." If Halpern, carried away by the excitement of being interviewed on a real radio program, found himself fabricating stories about official U.S. government music research foundations, this can be forgiven; but to include it in his book shows that he means to influence his readers with bald-faced lies. Such a tactic is at least unethical.

Does Halpern believe that the word "experiment" in a comment bestows scientific validity upon it? After muddling through a response to Don West's query on whether he had done any experiments with music, Halpern arrives at the heart of the matter. "Since that time," Halpern reports, referring to his days in college, "I have continued to conduct ongoing, 'subjective' experiments and 'listening tests' with people who attend my workshops and seminars. And of course I watch—and listen—when I go to a concert, or even to a supermarket, to observe how people react to the sounds around them."[2] Halpern truly believes that watching people in a supermarket is an experiment, and, as his books and lectures are replete with references to experiments and research, we must be skeptical of any comment Halpern makes that relies even in part on a so-called experiment, research, or test.

Halpern's *sole* experimental experience is reported in the chapter called "Experimentation" of his *Tuning the Human Instrument*:

Reflecting on previous experiments, I was struck by two main areas of conceptual myopia. For one thing, these earlier investigations had used solely physiological or psychological tests that failed to incorporate a holistic sense of the total human organism: We are not either a mind or a body. . . .

Music, as pure vibration and wavelength, has enormous potential in therapy, healing, and in effecting changes in personal and cultural consciousness. I knew intuitively that there are definite combinations of tones and intervals that can be used to maximize this positive potential, and my experiments were designed to find out what they were. When early pilot studies had shown that people were aesthetically turned off by a purely mechanical tone, subsequent experiments were limited to "music": So far as the people were concerned, if it weren't listenable, they wouldn't use it.[3]

Halpern would not use a physiological or psychological test to gauge his results, by his own admission. He neglects to explain what the alternative testing method could measure if not a physiological or psychological effect; but this is a minor difficulty compared to how Halpern tested what he "intuitively" knew about tones and intervals. Halpern admits that his early subjects were "turned off" by extramusical tones, so he stopped testing in this manner. In other words, Halpern decided not to use tones and intervals to test whether tones and intervals outside of a musical context can heal. One must question how he can possibly test the effectiveness of extramusical intervals if he doesn't have at least one segment of the test devoted to extramusical intervals. What Halpern does is simply ignore his own hypothesis, measure "Kirlian auras," and then claim that the presence of augmented auras has significance even though he never explains how auras are supposed to be used to evaluate his hypothesis. Though Halpern's "experiment" fails to test his hypothesis, he nevertheless reports,

In terms of their "dominant awareness" after listening to the Positive Affect Meditation tape, 100 percent of the subjects reported a response such as: "A very relaxed, meditative feeling"; "I felt like I was floating"; "Fantastic"; "It got me high." Nothing of this intensity was mentioned by the control group: "Moderately relaxing" was a response characteristic of 50% ("Just like most classical music.") 30% admired the pianist's technique, and 20% were bored by the selection.

In the answer to whether the selection had a more noticeable effect than most music: PAM and control, respectively, (100%, 20%). On the question of familiarity with the style: (25%, 100%). On the question of enjoyment of the music: (95%, 20%). Regarding the subjects' explanation of the effect, 100% of the experimental group mentioned the "unusual" nature of the rhythm: "It seemed to come in waves; I felt freedom to drift because I could not anticipate what would come next" was a characteristic response. Of the control selection, 80% reported no special effect: "Just like any other classical piece." (The other 20 percent noted that that selection was one of their favorites.)[4]

If much of this seems unclear, be warned that reading the entire chapter will not clarify anything but Halpern's inability to conduct a scientific experiment. Nevertheless, Halpern uses this "experiment" as proof of nearly everything he claims in lectures, books, and interviews. Barbara Anne Scarantino, in her book *Music Power*, decodes Halpern's experiment, though with some revisions (suggesting that she may have heard a lecture by Halpern on his experiment). She writes,

> In his fascinating book, *Tuning the Human Instrument,* Halpern describes his research. . . . Halpern designed the first experiments back in 1973 that involved both GSR (galvanized skin response), biofeedback, and Kirlian photography. . . . He and a team of associates played music for test subjects that had been classified by the *National Music Therapy Association* as being highly relaxing and meditative (such as "Liebestraum No. 3" by Liszt). They also used some music that Halpern himself had been working on aimed specifically at achieving relaxation ("Spectrum Suite"), and compared the test subjects' responses to these compositions.
>
> The results demonstrated that Halpern's music was far more conducive to actual physiological relaxation than the classical pieces, and the Kirlian images obtained with "Spectrum Suite" paralleled the results of studies that involved meditation and healing.
>
> Of course, Halpern composes his music specifically to be beneficial to your health and primarily to relax you. Most music, however, is

created for aesthetic (or monetary) reasons. This doesn't mean it is good or bad. It simply means that music that is truly beneficial to one's health and well-being does not come about by chance. It must contain the right elements so that the body involuntarily responds in a healthful, positive way, without mental suggestions or anticipation of a desired result.[5]

In *Sound Health,* his second book, Halpern's research takes yet another form. Halpern's experiment metamorphoses to suit any contention or hypothesis he is currently promoting. Testing organizations go through a metamorphosis in each retelling as well. In *Tuning the Human Instrument,* there appears the "Relaxation Research Foundation" an arm of the "U.S. Surgeon General's Office." In *Music Power* the "U.S. Surgeon General's office" is replaced by the fictitious "National Music Therapy Association" (or NMTA), and in *Sound Health* the "Relaxation Research Foundation" metamorphosizes into the "Psychotronic Research Institute." The Psychotronic team reported that Liszt's "Liebestraum No. 3" was rated by the subjects (yes, the subjects, not the U.S. Surgeon General's office or the NMTA) as "highly relaxing, soothing, and meditative," but Halpern claims that the subjects were all wrong. "The scientific equipment detected a high level of non-relaxed brain activity."[6] What equipment is he talking about? EEGs? CAT scans? No. "Kirlian photography." Kirlian photographs of the head? No, the fingers. A question that I cannot answer is why Halpern feels it necessary to refer at all to this continuously metamorphosizing research study when he has so many other nonexistent experiments to report.

When Don West asks Halpern how he justifies his color-tone-chakra congruency chart, Halpern refers to research with "thousands" of people. "How do you know that this correlation is correct?" asks West.

Empirically, it works! In my research I have come across a number of other systems, and have tried out, in experimental situations, other ways of relating the colors and tones. Some of these made people sick, others made it seem like a five-minute song lasted over half an hour. On the basis of feedback from thousands of people related to this seven-member system (7 tonal keynotes, 7 colors, 7 chakras) we know that this is a balanced set of stimuli that seems to allow for a consecutive stimulation of the areas of the body in a harmonically upward sweep ("the escalator effect"), terminating at the crown of the head.

The amount of negative reports that we have received can be counted on one hand. These usually come from individuals who subscribe to a specific religious sect. One other comment came from a 72-year-old woman, who sent me a clipping stating that the waltz is the only true music. She also said that Lawrence Welk is a reincarnation of Richard Strauss. Frankly, I can't believe that any composer could regress so far in one lifetime.[7]

Tangentially, I point out that I suspect that the seventy-two-year-old woman did not claim Welk as the reincarnation of Richard Strauss. She probably said, "Strauss," meaning Johann Strauss, the waltz king, not Richard Strauss whose few waltzes, I believe, have never been performed by Mr. Welk's band, assuming that Welk did not perform "Das Tanzlied" from *Also Sprach Zarathustra*.

Halpern's confusion regarding the scientific method is demonstrated in his comment: "For those of you who missed the newspaper articles, there are already companies in Texas and California who are using GSR [galvanic skin response] as a means of objectifying the advertised hype of a record 'to get the juices flowing.' "[8] Newspaper articles are not appropriate sources for judging the objective reliability of galvanic skin response machines (lie detectors).

Tabloid Science

Corinne Heline also looked in newspapers to bear testimony to her vision. She quotes from a newspaper article about the work of Margaret Anderton, whose "findings are so completely in harmony with the teachings of occultism . . . that we herewith quote from a published interview given by

Miss Anderton to the press."[9] In fact, the article is not an interview, but rather a third-person narrative in which Anderton is quoted. The article states that "tests" have proven that "certain pitches or harmonic combinations have a certain bodily effect. At present the effect on the throat of a certain chord in a certain key is being investigated, and it may prove to be of help in dealing with paralysis of the jaw."[10] The article fails to identify the test takers, the parameters, or the results. The only research identified is a thought experiment by Anderton, who says, "I had often thought about it, but it was crystallized for me one night after a concert when a man came to me in a state of great excitement and asked me why he had seen a certain color around the piano all the time that I was playing a certain composition."[11] Heline often cites newspaper articles and theosophical publications as scientific evidence for her occult beliefs.

A search through any newspaper will reveal that our daily periodicals (not even mentioning the lunatic fringe weeklies) do not maintain scientific fact-checkers on staff. An August 12, 1990, item plucked out of the *Tennessean* reveals the ignorance daily paraded as scientific fact. In an article headlined "Computers Bug Women, Study Finds," subheadlined "High Frequency Tone Doesn't Affect Men," a reporter basks in physiological/acoustical ignorance reporting a Grand Canyon–sized error in the easily disprovable statement that "men generally cannot hear above 15 kHz, while women can hear up to 18 kHz." Nothing in this statement approaches tested and commonly known acoustical and physiological fact. In addition, the procedure as reported in this article reveals that no research was actually done comparing men to women, only women to women. Despite these immense flaws, this article may become the linchpin to the next New Age music healing theory.[12]

Newspaper articles are simply unsuitable sources for scientific data. There is no rigorous screening involved in newspaper writing, which is why newspapers are filled with pseudoscientific gibberish. Much New Age research has the flavor of newspaper science reporting, fantasy mixed with nostalgic reverence for the tried and untrue. Halpern reports:

The moon also releases a high percentage of ultraviolet rays. Our modern society is "moonlight deprived." This is due, in no small measure, to artificial lighting—and dangerous city streets. To further enhance your quota of ultraviolet light, you can therefore expose yourself to more *moonlight*. There, you see: an ecologically sound excuse to go on a moonlight stroll. Although some people are hypersensitive to the energy of the full moon, it appears that moonlight deprivation during the rest of the month may cause health imbalance and psychic diseases for many other people, all of which probably goes unnoticed.[13]

The moon is not a radiant body. Any ultraviolet light it reflects is derived from sunlight and it would therefore be more realistic to receive this ultraviolet therapy during the day. Halpern does not seem to comprehend that "moonlight" is a poetic simplification of what is reflected sunlight.

Reflective of his own misunderstanding of the "scientific method," Halpern reads into the unscientific works of others the same scientific facade he perceives in his own. In *Sound Health*, Halpern and Savary report, "Dr. John Diamond, reporting in his book, *Your Body Doesn't Lie*, has scientifically observed groups of people listening to different recordings of the opening of the third movement of Beethoven's Ninth Symphony. If I play a performance of Beethoven's Ninth conducted by Furtwangler, I will see almost within seconds that the entire group is breathing synchronously, all their chests seem to be moving in unison."[14]

In fact, Diamond does no research. His books are collections of anecdotes and opinions. In *The Life Energy in Music*, Diamond writes, "According to popular tradition, women have a different sense of time. What I have learned from my study of female conductors has led me to the same conclusion."[15] There is pop psychology pablum throughout everything Diamond offers, but his "studies" amount to nothing more than going to concerts and annoying female conductors. "All female conductors I have tested—now over twenty of them—have high life energy whereas only a small percentage of male conductors have."[16] Diamond offers no explanation of how he tests the women, nor whether he has actually "tested" any male conductor. "It seems obvious that it is much easier for a woman to be a high energy conductor. This I believe is a biological reality. It is somehow easier for the female to submit to and transmit the pulse, perhaps because it is more in keeping with her psychophysiology."[17] It is obvious that Diamond is just tossing around some psychobabble in lieu of research. "Most female conductors do not like to hear me say this. They want to be regarded as equals with the males. They believe that there is no sex difference in conducting. My results show that there is. . . . It is a tragedy to find such high energy female conductors being forced to conduct mediocre orchestras."[18]

No wonder the female conductors do not like to hear Diamond's chauvinist fantasies: it is prejudice such as Diamond's that keeps female conductors chained to mediocre orchestras. "What of female instrumentalists? Here the difference does not apply. I am unable to explain this adequately and any reason I gave at this stage of investigation would be simply a guess. And what of female composers? Yes, we find that they also tend to be of high energy, confirming our theory that the genesis of music is in the feminine aspect of nature."[19]

Diamond attributes the lack of "important compositions written by women over the centuries, to "childrearing and mothering," which, he states, "reduc[es] or even eliminat[es] the need to compose."[20]

Deltoid Testing

Diamond's "scientific" research methods consist of two dubious techniques: "Respiratory Energy Spontaneous Pulsation" and "Deltoid Strength Testing." The latter consists of the tester pushing on the subject's arm to see if it is "weak" or "strong" in relation to whatever the tester is testing. This worthless technique, which shows only that a person's outstretched arm cannot resist a modest downward force, has been adopted by New Age conmen of sundry trades.

Diamond uses his Deltoid Testing Technique to assert his negative feelings about rock 'n' roll music. In 1979, Diamond claimed to have tested twenty thousand pieces of music with this dubious system.

> I have found only two instances in classical music that produce muscle weakness. One is at the conclusion of Stravinsky's *Rite of Spring* and the other at the conclusion of Ravel's *La Valse*... of the well over 20,000 records of all types of music that I have tested, only one other passage has caused the subject's indicator muscle to go weak, and that is one short segment of Haitian voodoo drumming. Nowhere else.
>
> Thus, this debilitating effect, which has come to be known as the Diamond Effect, is almost exclusively present in modern popular music. As far as my investigations can discern, it first emerged in the early sixties. Since then this beat has progressed until it is now well represented in the Top Ten of any week.[21]

Diamond precedes Halpern in the area of self-proclaimed eponymous "effects" with the pitiful attempt to engineer the entrance of his name into the English language. (Recall the "Halpern Effect.") Diamond also precedes several other New Age music healers in his Ravel-bashing, though what Ravel did to merit this widely held disesteem among music healers I am at a loss to explain. Perhaps it is because Ravel had a sense of humor and was able to impart this in his music. Or perhaps it is because Ravel managed to scoop other New Age composers by composing the twentieth century's answer to the Pachelbel Canon in D, viz: Bolero. As for Stravinsky's *Rite of Spring* causing muscle weakness in the arms or anywhere, this is certainly contradicted in the well-known report of its riot-provoking premiere, in which audience members participated in fisticuffs and general mayhem. An anecdotal report of this premiere has it that one member of the audience busied himself by pounding on the head of a listener directly in front of him, perhaps an early primitive version of Diamond's Deltoid Testing Technique.

Diamond has found that Bach's *Goldberg Variations* "relieves insomnia" and that Bach is feminine, as opposed to Beethoven, who is masculine.[22] Diamond analyzes Beethoven's "life energy" in a completely haphazard, superficial manner. He reports that the "Biological Harmonics research program of the Institutes [*sic*]" concluded that "in every case in which we have tested Beethoven's rejected sketches they have been of much lower energy than the final ones chosen. (His judgment in this was incredibly accurate.) This would also seem to indicate that it was only at the very last stages of composition that the determiner of the energy level, the pulse, was finally injected into the music."[23]

Is this not the same as saying that you always find a lost object in the last place you look? Of course Beethoven's rejected sketches are inferior to his final ones. That is what the process of composition is about. What do Beethoven's rejected sketches have to do with his life energy, anyway? How did they test his life energy? There is no explanation offered regarding the testing process. I wonder how Diamond convinced the West German government to allow him to exhume Beethoven's body and then, how the "life energy" of Beethoven's body could have been appropriately tested some century and a half after its burial.

But in an appendix at the end of Diamond's book that contains this "study" are the instructions for the three test procedures Diamond's institute uses to test "life energy." They are the "Standard Deltoid Test, " the "Thymus Test, " in which the Standard Deltoid Test is used, and the "Umbilicus Test," which also employs Standard Deltoid Test.

Diamond's second research technique is testing for "Respiratory Energy Spontaneous Pulsation." This means that at a concert, "with a high energy performer nearly everyone will be breathing in unison, as if the entire concert hall, including the performer, is pulsating at one with the composer."[24] Diamond's assertion is ludicrous. All wind instrumentalists and singers must perfect specialized breathing techniques which most members of an audience would find difficult to duplicate for a minute, much less an entire concert. An audience breathing in unison with the solo horn player during a Mozart horn concerto would be streaming for the exits before the end of the first movement. Many opera audience members would need hospitalization after breathing in unison with Placido Domingo during a Puccini aria.

> Over the years we at the Institutes for the Enhancement of Life Energy and Creativity have tested some 25,000 recordings of Western classical and popular music as well as the ethnic music of many cultures. Using specific testing on listeners, we have been able to delineate the degree of life energy enhancing qualities of most composers, and even the changes of energy as their musical lives progress. We can also delineate the precise degree of life energy enhancing qualities of the performers on all instruments as well as singers and conductors.
>
> The test is a purely objective test. There is nothing subjective about it. For the first time criticism is taken out of the realm of "I like it" or "I don't like it" or "It makes me feel good." This tests what it does physiologically.[25]

That Diamond claims objectivity for this test is evidence of a purposeful deceitfulness on his part. He counts on the gullibility of his reader (and their minimal observational abilities) not to demand proof. Assuming that of those twenty-five thousand recordings the average duration of each recording is a mere five minutes, then he has accumulated $2,083\frac{1}{3}$ hours of testing, or 260 eight-hour days of playing the music in the "Institute's" studio to a test audience, all of whose members are breathing in unison. How gullible does Diamond believe his readers are? By that, I mean his average readers. Halpern and Savary apparently believe in Diamond's research as legitimate.

> One of the problems with much of rock and pop music is its standard rhythm, what is called the "stopped-anapestic rhythm"—a "short-short-long-pause" pattern. This stopped-anapestic rhythm tends to confuse the body and weaken the muscles. Among hundreds of persons tested by

behavioral kinesiologist Dr. John Diamond, 90 percent registered an almost instantaneous loss of two-thirds of their muscle strength when they heard this beat. Interestingly, this often happens even when the listener likes the music.[26]

Reliance on Diamond's research is a major element in Halpern's oeuvre, as is his insistence that people just should not be trusted to make their own decisions about what music they should listen to (and his fanatical fear of anapestic rhythm.)

> The pop sound culture has invaded not only our homes and restaurants, but fitness centers as well. The problem is that the music people are using to exercise with or dance to often employs the stopped-anapestic rhythms that have actually been shown to weaken the strength of the muscles. Such music throws off muscular coordination and confuses the brain. The net result is that it will be even harder for you to learn tricky aerobics movements because the music itself may be confusing.[27]

The Man Who Heard Off the Scale

Halpern's belief that we should not listen to music we enjoy or find relaxing is founded in his belief that we do not have the "proper hearing apparatus." He says, "In a very real sense, then, at the core of our physical existence, we are composed of 'sound.' If we had the proper hearing apparatus, we might even be able to hear our own "harmony." Sensing this biological symphony at the cellular level is beyond the range of most of us."[28] When Halpern writes that the biological symphony of our cells is "beyond the range of most of us," he means us to understand that it is not beyond his range. In his 1988 Eastern Kentucky University lecture, Halpern described his first audiology test:

> But what I found out is that, not only did I hear that kind of music, but as they played up and down the scale with the little tones, I heard every-

thing that they played, and they said that if I had any hearing defects it was beyond their range of testing. I heard beyond their machines. And apparently there aren't too many people who did that. This was at Stanford University, and ten years later when I went back for a follow-up, the doctor, as I walked in the door, said, "You're the guy that heard off the scale." So I understood that there was something a little different, perhaps, about my apparatus.[29]

Halpern believes that he should serve as music arbiter of the world because of his superior hearing abilities. He wants us to believe that he is capable of showing us the true musical path to health because he is superior to us in regard to hearing, and that we normal people are not capable of much discretion in our musical choices. His music is scientifically proven to be perfect. Of his *Spectrum Suite* Halpern declares,

> First and foremost, the most noticeable response to this music is one of deep relaxation. . . . The relaxation is working on both the physiological as well as the psychological level. By so doing, the body is allowed to express its own inner nature and higher harmonics of functioning because of the degree of bio-rhythmic entrainment that goes on between the several main energy centers and oscillating systems in the body. It is this bio-entrainment and harmonization of the energy centers that allows us as individuals to tap into our Deep Self, which is finally scientifically recognized as having direct roots and vibrational connections with the earth and the cosmos. . . . The beauty of this music is that it works automatically and effortlessly.[30]

Halpern seems to imply the same easy path to enlightenment as do the distributors of subliminal tapes. In fact, Halpern has recently jumped on the subliminal tape bandwagon.

> We didn't get a chance to talk much about subliminals. There is another series that I have. These have gold covers. These are the only ones that

have subliminals. They use music that sounds like music on the other Anti-Frantic Series and using music as a carrier wave in which we imbed positive and uplifting statements. For people involved in pain control and other things I'll share with you there is a great deal of success beyond even what we had with *Spectrum Suite* and *Comfort Zone* by adding affirmations that suggest to the subconscious of the listener that, for instance that your body can secrete the proper hormones, the proper chemicals, to decrease pain, that your body knows how to heal itself to encourage and support it to heal itself. Speaking directly to the brain is definitely one of the areas that we're going to be seeing a lot more work.[31]

In the same lecture Halpern again explains why people should not be allowed to choose their own music to enjoy in yet another restatement of his classic "experiment."

Seventy-six point one percent of the people said that "Liebestraum No. 3" by Liszt was the most relaxing piece of music they knew of. Now, that was before *Spectrum Suite* [laughter]. What we've found doing the research is, number one, that it did not relax people within a hundred-fold of what *this* music was doing. Now, interestingly, this was true even if, and we have several people who swore up and down sometimes quite vociferously, that the music was relaxing them; from which I deduced a major observation and a major truth; that many many people don't know a relaxation state if it came up and bit them on the elbow.[32]

Halpern's positions oscillate endlessly. He writes his music intuitively; no, he writes it based on scientific experiments. There is a specific human harmonic; there are many individual frequencies for each organ. In one book Halpern attacked Muzak but in one lecture he even went so far as to refer to his own work as a kind of Muzak. This condition of constant wavering is not Halpern's alone. He shares it with many of his brethren. It can be heard in the music healers' pointed attacks on Western music and culture while they persevere in composing only in equal temperament and Western style. It can be seen in their attempts to defend their music as "science" while simultaneously attacking science as fascistic Western blindness. One can recognize the panic in frenzied attempts to reconstruct acoustics to validate their compositional techniques, which are not in the least connected to their music-making.

What is it that compels music healers to create such bomphilogy to rationalize their music? Beethoven never felt compelled to defend his advanced "New Age" harmonies and structure with fabulous theories. He just wrote. There it is, the answer to the question: Beethoven. Beethoven, Mozart, Bach, Stravinsky, Wagner, Brahms, Mahler, even Liszt (maybe especially Liszt). These titans cast their shadows over New Age music healer/composers with such ecliptic menace that they feel compelled to scurry about denying them. No treatise on the scientific rightness of a piece will etch for it a place in our hearts. No attack on the male-dominated nineteenth century will erase a single note of Beethoven. No veridical analysis of the evil personality of Wagner will alter the power of Wagner to affect us. Steven Halpern argues against what he perceives as a "tyranny of tradition" when he criticizes music therapist Helen Bonny's use of classical music in her method, Guided Imagery and Music. It upsets Halpern that music therapists of Bonny's stature find his music lacking.

> Many of the ideological patron saints of the movement such as Helen Bonny . . . get stuck at a certain point in the compilation of literature. Helen Bonny, which I was reading, commits a very strange sin of quoting a critic from the *New York Times* who admittedly knows nothing about New Age music and yet says some of the typically very, very negative things about it. . . . [Bonny] is someone who should know better; that there is a lot more to the music than just something that's boring.[33]

Halpern's reference to his own music as boring should not go unnoticed; but he prefers to attack tradition rather than hone his skills so that his music might not be "just something that's boring."

Howard Richman also describes his own music in less than sterling adjectives. "It is not all necessarily pleasant to the ear," he warns in his promotional materials. In an interview with Ruth Marks Richman explained that people listening to his music "may not like the sound of it or the feeling it gives them."[34] Richman does not challenge classical music, which is an attitude Halpern might be well advised to emulate. In his 1988 Eastern Kentucky University lecture Halpern launched himself into a tirade against classical music, reality, and New Age music.

> One of the things that I feel that my work has demonstrated over the last twenty years is that certainly all music or most of the music that we are taught about in school is Western European music, and there's a lot more to music than just some little black dots written on white paper by dead European composers [applause and laughter]. . . . I've had to deal with a lot of people who have misunderstood a lot of my own compositions over the years. There is a rhythm even in some of my nonrhythmic music. . . . But, it's rhythm of alpha waves, it's rhythm of theta waves, it's rhythm of the yogic deep breath. If you listen to the spaces between the notes you'll find that there is an organization that goes on in my compositions that's not just by bar lines. And it's not just by heartbeat lines, but heartbeats of the composer, performing, recording artist who has gotten himself into a composed state. So I am playing my own nervous system. I am playing and working on that aspect of rhythm. Playing my own biorhythms. . . . A fundamental principle is that the composer must compose him or herself. So this is the musician's oath, the Pythagorean oath, possibly parallel to the Hippocratic oath, "Physician, heal thyself." Something that most people, even who work in New Age music, don't pay attention to.[35]

Halpern's self-aggrandizement and advertisement does not sit well with several of his brethren. David Tame believes that a deficient concept provides the foundation stone for the music of Steven Halpern. . . . And what, to Steven Halpern, is the purpose of his music? In all of his talks and writings the same criterion keeps appearing by which all music, it seems, should be judged: that music should be "healing." Again, hardly a despicable idea at first sight. However, the term "healing," as used and understood by many, is frequently as far from the genuine meaning of the word as is the "peace" of the Kremlin or the "love" of the sexually permissive.[36]

Tame asserts that Halpern does not appreciate that healing music should

include tonal art which helps to perfect and align the totality of man's being. In this sense, classical and all genuinely good music is certainly healing: healing in the word's truest and fullest sense, as a harmonizer and improver of each aspect of man's being—physical, emotional, mental and spiritual. In his talks, however, Halpern has never seemed particularly enthusiastic about classical music. After all, works such as Elgar's tremendous *Pomp and Circumstance* marches or Verdi's *Aida* are hardly "healing" in the sense of being soporific, marijuana-music.[37]

Tame is most lucid when expressing his immense lack of respect for New Age music. He writes,

If a new and better era awaits humanity, its successful manifestation will certainly require men and women of *true spirituality*—which is to say, men and women of both mystical heart *and practical mind.* Active and capable intellects will be an essential. It demands little foresight to realize that planet earth will never be improved by sitting back in a cloud of incense or by falling asleep to an electronic sound-massage. Is, then, the music of Stephen Halpern [*sic*], Steve Hillage and others truly New Age music? Does it raise our hearts with inspiration to be self-sacrificing? Does it divinely organize our minds? Does it impel us to awaken to the challenges of the hour in the world at large, as, directly or indirectly, any genuine New Age music must? Not when it is an impulsive chaos of jazz. Not when it is over-electronic and divorced from human feelings. Not when, as it so often is, it is a synthetic mist of psychedelic miasma.[38]

Unfortunately, Tame's lucid philosophical argument against Halpern and his ilk soon changes into another Blavatsky-inspired screed. Tame seems to develop amnesia in regard to his praise of great classical composers when he recommends that tone poems by Norman Thomas Miller should be regarded as true New Age music. "Working from a background of the teachings of the Great White Brotherhood . . . N. T. Miller's most important work to date is *The Call of Camelot,* a thirty minute tone poem of unique and scorching spirituality . . . there could hardly be a composition more picturesque—and even photographic—in the clarity of the visions which it offers to the attuned listener."[39]

Tame chooses to sanctify composers whose music he likes while vilifying the composers whose work he dislikes. He vituperatively attacks Tchaikovsky and Mussorgsky and obsequiously worships Miller and Wagner. Tame promotes cults of personality, a belief that only "great" men can write great music. Thus, Tame has more in common with Halpern than he might care to admit: the fundamental, and inherently flawed, conclusion that some music is objectively good and some music is objectively bad. Halpern and Savary write that there is music that "transcends personal tastes, a music to which the nervous system wants to dance, a music that does not require intellectual analysis or emotional involvement."[40] Not surprisingly, they identify this music as Halpern's *Spectrum Suite.*

Misconstruing Classical Music

Classical music is a stumbling block to more New Age music healers than Halpern and Tame. John Diamond, too, is ill at ease in this milieu. In volume 2 of *Life Energy in Music* Diamond regales us with many stories regarding classical music and healing. Reporting on a recording session that a recording engineer misguidedly allowed Diamond to attend, Diamond writes,

> In the two days of this recording session I heard considerable discussion, mainly from Bill, as to their sixteenth notes and technical matters like that. But I never once heard any mention of the important qualities in music; of line, of gesture, of pulse, of meaning, of purpose, let alone of warmth, or love, or humanity. . . . I soon got the impression, which was continually reinforced over the two days, that I was hearing two technicians who really cared nothing for the music.[41]

Clearly Diamond does not understand that classical musicians are technicians, that they spend years of their lives training to build up technical skills which they must keep in fine condition through practice. Classical musicians spend years of their lives learning to play scales in a mechanical, even fashion. Robotic, inhuman precision is a necessary prerequisite for classical musicians from the last chair second violinist in the orchestra to the soloist. How do most keyboard players and conductors interpret Bach? Precise, even, and with the smallest amount of dynamic differentiation necessary. This severely unexpressive interpretation is what allows Bach's music to move us to the depths of our souls. A group of weeping, crying, instrumentalists expressing their individuality would destroy entirely any meaning in one of Bach's Brandenburg concerti.

Diamond complains that he "never once heard any mention of the important qualities in music; of line, of gesture, of pulse, of meaning, of purpose, let alone of warmth, or love, or humanity," at the recording session. On the contrary, I suspect he heard, he just didn't understand. No mention of line, Diamond says. But the conductor probably was saying that he wanted a passage in the strings played beginning with an upbow preceding measure 150, followed by two down bows and an upbow again preceding measure 151. There was "line." "Of gesture" Diamond noted nothing, but he also probably made nothing of the conductor's likely remarks of "sul tasto" or his barked command to the horns to play softer. "Of pulse" he complains that nothing was said, but then he does not understand that the conductor is speaking eloquently of pulse with his baton and the instrumentalists are constantly aware of it. Nothing "of meaning, of purpose . . . of warmth, or love, or humanity," laments Diamond, but Diamond is just unlearned. It is all there for him to see and hear, but he is looking in the wrong place and worse, he is listening for the wrong sounds. It is not the words, it is the music that carries the meaning. Say all you want about humanity, but if you are not able to play your part correctly, you are not able to express anything.

> Every art is wearisome, in the learning of it, to the untaught and unskilled. Yet things that are made by the arts immediately declare their use, and for what they were made, and in most of them is something attractive and pleasing. And thus when a shoemaker is learning his trade it is no pleasure to stand by and observe him, but the shoe is useful, and moreover not unpleasing to behold. And the learning of a carpenter's trade is very grievous to an untaught person who happens to be present, but the work done declares the need of the art. But far more is this seen in music, for if you are by where one is learning, it will appear the most painful of all instructions; but that which is produced by the musical art is sweet and delightful to hear, even to those who are untaught in it.[42]

Two thousand years after Epictetus made these comments to Arrian, it still holds true, and Diamond may not have spoken of a lack of warmth, or love, or humanity had he read and appreciated it. The extent of Diamond's misunderstanding of music is revealed in his "research." In writing about Berlioz and Beethoven he cites Hugh McDonald, but this is just a citation from the *New Grove Dictionary of Music and Musicians*, not useful for more than the most elementary information on these composers. Diamond's books are compendiums of shallow musical insights and anecdotal reports of Diamond's therapeutic cures using his personal views of music to implement them.

Alfred Tomatis attempts to legitimize his "Tomatis Effect" with classical music, though his Tomatis Effect is, supposedly, purely acoustic, in other words, extramusical. His exclusive use of Mozart is oddly distorted because he filters out the lower frequencies. Patricia Joudry notes,

> The music was recognizably Mozart, though Mozart would have had a fit. The violin concertos, symphonies and chamber pieces all started out normally, except for occasional soft hissing sounds. Then, imperceptibly, the lower sounds began giving way to the strings. After a time even the strings were clinging to the rafters. It was strange, eerie, and perversely pleasing. Yet I wondered. It just didn't seem possible that sitting here listening to squeaky music for three hours was going to relieve me of anything but thirty-six dollars. (By now the fee is considerably higher, all low prices having been filtered out everywhere.)[43]

That it is the nature of music to mean different things to its listeners seems to have evaded music healers. They parade their own unique responses as if they should ring a bell in everyone's soul, and are blind to the fact that their revelations are not universal, but simply personal.

David Tame, in *The Secret Power of Music,* unveils a chart that gives "examples of music which correctly energize the chakra by expressing the divine qualities of the ray," as well as "musical styles which particularly pervert the correct functioning of the chakra."[44] Tame derives this chart from the work of Elizabeth Clare Prophet, a self-proclaimed contemporary prophet living in a cult community originally started by her deceased husband, Mark. Prophet and Tame suggest that symphonies energize the crown chakra, while piano concerti energize the next lower chakra. The throat chakra is energized by marches (such as *Pomp and Circumstance* Nos. 1 and 4) and the heart chakra is energized by waltzes and harp music. The root chakra, they say, is energized by "early American patriotic pieces and the rhythms of Indian classical music." The perverting influences are "jazz, computer music (the 'new music'), rock vocals, also folk-rock vocals; foxtrot, tango and the 'jazz waltz,' blues, that which is *called* 'soul' music, and voodoo and rock rhythm" in successive order from the crown to the root chakra (emphasis original).[45] Tame may view classical music as beneficial, though his simplistic renderings of it (that is, "symphonies" for the crown chakra) are embarrassing; but Tame's fear of rock music is comic. He suggests that "the best critique on all aspects of rock" is David Noebel's *The Marxist Minstrels: A Handbook on Communist Subversion of Music*, which Tame describes as a "labour of love by a dedicated moral researcher."[46]

Manly Hall has also confused his personal predilections for objective truth.

> Experience shows that a certain type of music has the broadest appeal to every class of audience. . . . By trial and error it has been learned that jazz has little or no therapeutic value. If this seems to be an attack upon a popular music form, the outraged disciples of syncopation can take heart in the thought that grand opera is no better. Jazz is a stimulant and an irritant and so are all compositions featuring broken rhythms, dissonances, and exaggerated tempo. Most operatic selections require too much listening, as well as highly trained acceptance and appreciation.
>
> Further research has eliminated vocal music. Words do not always broadcast clearly, and the mind becomes actively intrigued and instinctively listens. Intense rhythms fatigue those who hear them and cause a positive reaction such as the effort to keep time with the feet or by nodding the head. Semiclassical music, featuring persuasive melodies and old familiar tunes—sometimes slightly nostalgic—is the most successful. A pleasant melodic line, carried mostly in the strings and not noticeable in the brass percussions, was found to be universally acceptable, fulfilling the old doctrine of Pythagoras.[47]

Here Hall confuses "popular" with "beneficial." It is difficult to criticize his comments, including his invocation of Pythagoras, because they are so touchingly misguided.

Peter Michael Hamel, who is opposed in philosophy if not musical preference to Hall, and in agreement with Tame, warns of the insidious influence of "beat music."

> In such a situation it is understandable that music too has become a mere commercial drug. On the one hand we have the sentimentality of the tear-jerkers in the bars, on the other the aggressiveness of the mindless Rock music in the "drug-dives." The identification-mechanism linking music to listener is, as I indicated at the outset, clearly recognisable: most music reflects and bolsters up the state of its clientele, their inner chaos, their private insecurity and loneliness. While the greater part of Pop music is produced under the influence of drugs, many so-called "session-musicians" of the Beat music industry are alcoholics.[48]

Nor is Hamel an admirer of classical music; he spews misconceptions about classical music and its composers. "Scriabin developed a mystical scale which is very close to the chromatic scales of the orient, and from which he derived in his numerous piano works, harmonic clusters that were literally unheard-of in his day."[49] Untrue and untrue. Hamel asserts that "Anton von Webern's twelve-note technique and the theories of the latter's pupil Rene Leibowitz [were] to become the basis of so-called Serial music."[50] Webern would have blushed in shame to see himself and his pupil described as the "basis" of serial music, when it was Webern's teacher, Schoenberg, who is its universally recognized father (with the only proviso being the rather slight influence of Josef Hauer). Webern's contribution to serialism is generally regarded as Klang-Farben melody, a technique he drew from Schoenberg's *Five Orchestral Pieces*. There is nothing else that Webern invented or described that he did not correctly attribute to Schoenberg's teachings.

Many who write about music from a New Age perspective must believe that those who read their scribblings are musically illiterate and incapable of aesthetic judgment on their own. Hal Lingerman's *Healing Energies of Music* is filled with Lingerman's opinions, his likes and dislikes; but Lingerman is not satisfied with conveying his musical tastes; he imparts an "objective" criticism that designates certain composers and their works as bad for your health. "Ravel's 'Bolero' is a very harmful piece of music which should be avoided," he writes.[51] I admit, it is not a great work, but it is difficult to accept its mediocrity as actually harmful.

Kay Gardner rarely discusses classical music, with the exception of Pachelbel's Canon. In her article, "On Composing Medical Music" Gardner accompanies her example of the passacaglia bass pitches from Pachelbel's misnamed Canon with the comment, "Why else in this age of social and technocratic anxiety is this three hundred year old composition, based upon an eight note chant, such a hit?"[52] Gardner's example, the bass, is as far from chant as a bass can get. In the eight intervals of the bass, only three are intervals of less than a perfect fourth. The leaps are completely uncharacteristic of chant. The example of chant Gardner gives, "nam myoho renge kyo," for instance, consists of six syllables sung to the same pitch.[53] No intervals, even of a second. The characteristics of Pachelbel's bass are so antithetical to the nature of chant that we can only assume that Gardner assumes that everything in music is chant, in which case, why pick on poor Pachelbel and his only claim to immortality?

In *The Music of Life*, Hazrat Inayat Khan states his disdain for music of more than one instrument, and notes a nonexistent trend towards "more natural" music.

> We can observe two principal tendencies in modern music. One is the tendency to make the music of our time more natural, and in that way to improve it. This can surely be developed more and more, as there will be a greater appreciation of solo music, for instance of the cello or the violin. Musicians will again go back to the ancient idea of one instrument playing or one voice singing at a time. When they again come to the full appreciation of this idea, they will reach the spiritual stage of

musical perfection. . . . The reason why two sounds are in conflict with each other is that however much they are tuned to one another, yet they are two, and that in itself is a conflict. There is another tendency that is working hand in hand with this one and is dragging music downward. Composers are not content with the chords that the great masters such as Mozart, Beethoven, or Wagner have used in their music, but they are inventing new chords, chords that tend to confuse thousands of listeners. . . . It will have an unconscious effect upon the nervous system of humanity; it will make people more and more nervous. As we often see that those who attend good concerts only go there out of vanity, they will accept any kind of music. But, as Wagner has said, noise is not necessarily music.[54]

With the exception of works for piano (which "has more than one voice") the masters he mentions always wrote for multiple instruments and voices. In addition, Beethoven and Wagner were both regarded as being discontented with the "chords" of their time periods. Wagner's *Tristan und Isolde* is notorious for its "Tristan chord," which was novel in its harmonic function; and Beethoven's blaring D naturals in the *Eroica* Symphony created a sonority unheard of at the time, not to mention the brash dissonant chord of the final movement of the *Ninth* Symphony (a B♭ major triad with a frightening A natural in the timpani and trumpets;) and Mozart's music is not without its unnerving chords, such as those that open the *Dissonant* Quartet. These are just a few of the more well-known examples. Khan fails to understand his examples and undermines any credence in his words with such nonsense as people preferring "the solo music."

"I have often thought," remarks Khan, "that if Scriabin, with his fine character and beautiful personality, had lived longer, he could have introduced a new strain of music into the modern world."[55] Well, as Khan admits to his fine character (which many other New Age music theorists would disagree with) and beautiful personality, could Khan not find any work of merit in the seventy-four published and nine unpublished works of Scriabin? Or did he acquire his fine character and beautiful personality only after Opus 74, immediately prior to his death? If his fine character and beautiful personality did not help him with the eighty-three prior works, how could it have helped with number eighty-four? (Incidentally, the opus numbers do not refer only to single pieces. As many as two dozen separate pieces are included under single opus numbers.)

British composer Cyril Scott relied upon by New Age music healers as their link to Steiner and Blavatsky, commented at length on classical composers, but most revealing of his writing is his racist stereotyping in his writing on Indian classical music.

> That Indian music affected chiefly the mind, we have endeavoured to show; furthermore, because it lacked in general those more energising elements of our varied Western music, we find that the people of India lack those elements also.... Inasmuch as their music lacked variety, lacked energy, lacked power, so have the Indians themselves as a race remained one-sided, inert and unequally balanced in character....
>
> Indian music has remained largely of the homophonic restricted type. An art so circumscribed, into which comes no novelty of idea, which, in short, does not progress, is apt to fade into insignificance. If music in the West had remained stationary, it, too, would have suffered a similar fate.
>
> As the love of music itself is often transmitted from parent to child or grandchild, is it not probable that the effects of that music upon character will also be transmitted? And if that music, as in India, has been passed on through scores of generations, will its effects not have become correspondingly intensified? If we admit this, we shall understand the characteristic lethargy of the Indian people.[56]

It must be agreed that the love of music is often transmitted from parent to child, but it is saddening to read Scott's ethnocentric racism placed in a central position in regard to the music of India.

R. J. Stewart is unique among music healers in that he seems to reject classical and all other music completely. Classical music "has a continual tendency towards degeneration, to devolution, and ossification."[57] One has to assume Stewart does not like it. Music that comes from "oral or folk traditions," he says, "has a tendency to become static and ultra-conservative." However, he notes that such music can be saved if not "divorced from the mainstream," which, however, he describes as no longer expressing "the voice of the people—unless we accept that the people merely require trivia and banality."[58] As far as can be determined from his writing, Stewart simply dislikes all music, other than "chanting" on healing pitches.

Part of New Age philosophy mirrored by many New Age music healers is a dissatisfaction with Western tradition. To fight Western tradition they leap to the conclusion that Eastern tradition must be diametrically opposed to Western, hence superior. Herein lies the rub. Both traditions are rigid. Both East and West share the same tendency—for spiritualism to become ritualism. The West has Christianity; the East, Buddhism. The West has the Hail Mary; the East, Hare Rama. Belief in a special status for Eastern philosophies is peculiarly racist. Are the Chinese inscrutable? No more so than the Swedish. In avulsing bits and pieces of Buddhist or Hindu or Egyptian or ancient Greek philosophy and science the New Age music healer ignores the real location of wisdom: contemporary science and their own artistic traditions. They take their shallow vision of Buddhism and transmogrify it into base trivialism. They make of Buddhism a toy, a trinket.

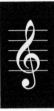

8. Testimonials: Right Conduct

Behold, the beginning of philosophy is the observation of how men contradict each other, and the search whence cometh this contradiction, and the censure and mistrust of bare opinion. And it is an inquiry into that which *seems*, whether it rightly *seems*, and the discovery of a certain rule, even as we have found a balance for weights, and a plumb line for straight and crooked. This is the beginning of philosophy.[1]

Quick Cures

At the heart of my objections to New Age music healing is my belief that most of its practitioners are not acting ethically. Those to whom are entrusted the health of others have an especial obligation to act ethically. There is a lesser quality of ethical misconduct in the newspaper astrologer than in the psychic charlatan that preys on individuals. There is a high level of ethical misconduct on the part of those persons who present themselves as healers under false pretenses and thereby hoodwink and endanger those who place their faith in them. If my book *seems* mean-spirited, it is less so than those it *discovers*. Perhaps it is less so because

251

Seeming, doth not for every man answer to Being; for neither in weights or measures doth the bare appearance content us, but for each case we have discovered some rule. . . . For this it is, that when it is discovered cureth of their madness those that mismeasure all things by *seeming* alone; so that henceforth, setting out from things known and investigated, we may use an organized body of natural conceptions in our several dealings.[2]

Claims of cures from music and sound treatments by music healers are evident throughout the literature on music healing, but what are we to make of healing through machines? "Somatron" and "Betar" are trade names for tables, not simple tables, but very elaborately designed couches. Somasonics, Inc., the Somatron company, sells one of its couches, the Athena 2000, for $7,000. Its least expensive somasonic couch, the Somatron Sound *Lounge*, is just $2,500. The sound lounge is practically made of speakers, so that you can listen to the music while being enveloped in it. The idea of the Somatron is innocuous, and Byron Eakin, the Tampa, Florida, oil painter, who designed the couch sells it without much hyperbole (a reserve that the Betar creators do not share.) Dimensional Sciences, Inc., sells the Betar, a more elaborate version of the Somatron. Unlike its softsell competitor, Somasonics, Dimensional Sciences has a histrionic and bizarre sales pitch. It begins, calmly and sanely enough, with "Some Reflections on the Healing Power of Sound, Language, and Music: A Report on the Betar Biological Scanning System." The material purports to be a reprint of a piece by Tom Kenyon, co-director of Acoustic Brain Research, who writes for Interdimensional Sciences, which is the same company as Dimensional Sciences. (They are located at the same address.) Kenyon's article is primarily a description of his work with Margo. "There was . . . something in my experience with Margo. In fact, I had experienced it with every person I had worked with where what I call *true healing* took place. This something was what many people call energy, a feeling that I felt when things were right, and often times my clients felt it too. We would sit together looking at each other ga-ga eyed. No words could describe it, and when we tried they were ridiculously trite."[3]

Kenyon (who is not a doctor) explains that Margo has cancer that is "spreading." Kenyon plays her "music I had chosen especially written with spacious silences between the lush phrases," but chooses not to identify the piece. He says he leads her on an "imaging process" with the music, guiding her "deeper into the fantasy, telling her to bring the energy . . . up into her spine where the cancer was most rampant. . . . When she opened her eyes she said, 'It's gone!' 'What's gone?' I asked. 'The pain.' "[4] Kenyon reports that Margo is still alive two years later, leading his reader, naturally, to assume that Margo has been cured of cancer through the use of the Betar Biological Scanning System. Kenyon's article refers to Tomatis, Ernst Rossi, and especially Peter Kelly, the "inventor" of the Betar.

I noticed that the most powerfully transforming sessions seemed to have the greatest amount of the *energy*. I tried to label it, work with it, read about it. And as a researcher I tried to figure out a way to document it.

The problem was that from a clinical standpoint it did not exist since it could not be measured. Write that up to science's arrogance if you wish. But going back to Pribram's point, in science, without something to measure, there is nothing to share.

In terms of the body's energy field, that is all beginning to change. There is much work going on around the world concerning the quantification or scientific measurement of the human energy field. I would like to discuss one of these major developments.

Tucked away in the gently rolling hills of Lakemont, Georgia, is a remarkable laboratory called Interdimensional Sciences. Interdimensional Sciences is headed by Peter Kelly, one of the most talented engineers and innovators I have ever met. Peter has developed, over the years, a system of Agricultural Radionics.[5]

Kenyon claims that Kelly has documented evidence that his system of "Agricultural Radionics" rids "fields of insect pests, increases yields, and so on, all without the use of pesticides."[6] Kenyon chooses not to burden us with any references to the "documented" evidence. Peter Kelly's agricultural work is but the tip of Kelly's iceberg of innovation. According to Kenyon, Kelly's greatest work is a psychoacoustic device called the Betar. The Betar is in part a geodesic dome in which the patient reclines on what Kelly calls a "Transduction Table." Speakers are placed around the table. These speakers, according to Kenyon again (Kelly is either too modest or too wise to say so himself), are in *"phase conjugation* which means that when one speaker pulses vibration to the body, the opposite speaker pulls the vibration to itself through the body."[7] Kenyon does not choose to explain how a speaker can pull vibration to itself through the body, because it is an utterly absurd claim. Speakers transmit, they do not suck. There is no device in existence that can suck sound out of anything. Would that there were so that people could defend themselves from boom-box carriers on the streets of our cities.

> Recently, the Betar entered a whole new realm. Again, using the scalar technology he developed for his Agricultural Radionics, Peter has developed a Biological Scanning System which has become part of the Betar. It picks up the energy field of the body within the 4–16 Hz range. There are no electrodes attached to the body. The scanning system reads the energy of the body from the *Transduction Table* within the Betar. It is not affected by music or electromagnetic fields. It reads the body, and only the body.
>
> Further, the system is linked with a computer which gives numeric and visual readouts of the energy. Remember what Karl Pribram said about quantification? We now have something to share.[8]

But does the Betar work? To answer the question one has to know what the question really is. The Betar cannot suck vibrations out of bodies through speakers or *any* apparatus. What it "measures" as output from the body is nothing. This is a bogus claim. You cannot measure a brain wave outside the skull without at least "an electrode." Kelly's machine, aside from its ability to broadcast music as any stereo system can, does nothing; but the Betar does cost $45,000 and is the best-publicized representative of the stereo couch concept. It is no crime to sell stereos for $45,000, but Kelly and Kenyon, intentionally or not, are certainly deceptive in their commentary. The definition of fraud, in the U.S. courts, includes intent, and I cannot document intent. In concluding his "Reprint" article, Kenyon notes: "With the Betar, we can show the Margos of the world how the energy fields of their bodies change in response to music therapy or Psychoacoustic sessions. . . . Finally, to those skeptical minds who doubt what they cannot see, I say, look again."[9]

I did look again, especially since Kelly was describing his work as music therapy, and this is what I found. Kelly, the inventor of the Betar, a high school graduate, started research in the field of "Radionics-Psychotronics" in 1970, shortly before becoming a student of someone he identifies in his resume as Swami Rama. A self-proclaimed pioneer in "psychotronic map dowsing," he was busy in 1977 "locating underwater pyramids in the Florida trench and various Atlantean artifacts of archaeological value." These accomplishments are not exactly believable, nor are they documented. In 1977 Kelly says he "discovered" the "correlation between diagrams of Chakra lotus petals and 'frequency' of Chakras." That's nice. Though he worked with T. G. Hieronymus, "an early radionics pioneer," Kelly notes that he has no current association with him (whoever he is.)[10] If these details of Kelly's life recall the paintings of Hieronymous Bosch, his writing is more like the art work of Arcimboldo. You have to stand far away from it to determine what it is Kelly is describing. And far away is the distance I would stay from Kelly and Kenyon and their quick cures on a $45,000 table that transmits and sucks vibrations from bodies. How is this music therapy? Where is the music? The therapy? The human contact?

The technique of "toning" was popularized in music-healing circles in the United States by Laurel Keyes. Keyes's toning originated in the faith-healing work of the Fransisters, a religious group Keyes founded in 1963. Keyes was inspired by her discovery of the benefits of toning to heal the world. She and the Fransisters received healing requests from all over the world and responded. Her scientific rationale for toning, Keyes explains, is based on the book *Radionics, Radiesthesia, and Physics,* by William Tiller of the Academy of Parapsychology and Medicine. "I do believe that Dr. Tiller has explained how it [toning] works in his paper on nodal points extending from a field. 'To be in resonance with any one of these points, is to be in resonance with the particular gland of the entity.' "[11] Keyes joins Kelly, Kenyon, and their Betar on the cancer-cure bandwagon with her toning technique.

> A dentist had a biopsy of an unhealed condition in his lip and found it positive. He made arrangements to have radiation treatment and plastic surgery. But . . . he postponed the treatment for 6 weeks. In the meantime his wife Toned for his condition and he Toned with her. . . .
>
> Within 10 days a scab fell off with tiny hair roots, shriveled, still attached to it. It was as though it had been dried up from the tips of the roots, outward, and "died" from the vibration of the Toning. No treatment was necessary. No scar was left. No recurrence of it after 6 years.
>
> Another case of skin cancer was that of a woman who had received radiation treatment for it. When it recurred in the same area less than two years later, she Toned. . . . After the first day she said the flesh became swollen and red and had every appearance of having had radiation. "It looked just as it had when I had X-ray treatments." Within a week it was normal again. No recurrence. No other treatment was needed.[12]

Toning, according to Keyes, can heal everything: cancer, diabetes, headaches. Keyes's most astonishing claim is that toning can heal without the presence of the subject that is being healed.

A teacher, whom we knew, had suffered a pain in his right arm and shoulder for weeks. In spite of medication it continued to grow worse. . . . It had made it impossible for him to write on the blackboard or raise his arm above his head.

We Toned for him, without his knowledge. That evening he was called and asked how he felt.

"The oddest thing happened today," he replied. "For no reason that I know of my arm felt better. I could write on the board, something I've not been able to do for a long time. I can't understand it. The pain is just gone. It's just a little sore but not stiff."

The soreness disappeared within a week and there was no more trouble with the arm. This young man was a very intellectual person and if he had known that we were trying to "heal" him, we were sure that his mind would have rejected it. Since he did not know, he was helped.[13]

With this sort of evidence, Keyes can claim to have cured anyone and everything. It defies reason that she did not even consider the fact that medication might have had something to do with this teacher's arm getting better. On the other hand, a young man with a sore arm who simply recovers as his own body heals itself, this is not world-shattering news. The anecdote is so silly and pointless that Keyes should think better of telling anyone this story, much less committing it to print.

I can comprehend Keyes's religiously based belief that prayer can heal. Keyes's prayer is accompanied by "toning," just as religious "healing" has been accompanied for centuries worldwide by the chanting shaman. But Keyes's belief that the positive effects of sound transcend physical barriers has a reverse side. What then of the evil wishes of people? Can they be communicated through the ether? What of bad concerts? Do they leave a negative residue?

But Keyes enlists science in her religious beliefs, and science and faith are mutually exclusive. Faith demands belief without evidence or proof. That is its definition. Science demands proof. This is not meant to condemn either science or faith, but to condemn the confusion created by mixing the two. The Catholic church has long recognized the importance of this separation, ever since the church recognized its error with Galileo. Cardinal Baronius wrote in the seventeenth century, "The intention of the Holy Ghost is to teach us how one gets to heaven, not how heaven goes."[14] Unfortunately, Baronius was dead before Galileo's trial and could not serve on the ecclesiastical jury.

Most New Age music healers have neglected to learn the lesson of the Catholic church, and instead use science to support beliefs not supportable and often antithetical to the scientific method. Sometimes they create scientific-sounding names for their techniques or organizations. Often they fail to mention the real source of their science, fearing, perhaps, that the revelation that their science is founded in the esoteric philosophy of Blavatsky or Steiner would prove injurious to their reputations.

Music healers must recognize that clients' diseases may be multifaceted, not subject to cure with simplistic, single-issue approaches. The music healer that believes that health can be obtained through a pitch or a tape of behavioral commands is offering little help to the individual whose illness affects a wide range of behaviors in himself *and* others. Is there a pitch that not only obliterates the alcoholic's dependency on alcohol, but also ameliorates the effects of the alcoholic's previous behavior on his familial relationships? In what way is the New Age model of healing, as represented by the New Age music healers, holistic?

Many New Age music healers talk a good game railing against impersonal models of medicine and therapy, but the practice of most music healing is extremely impersonal. This is obvious in the focus upon the machines, the tapes, the chakra systems; and if one explored the whole field of New Age healing (not just music healing) one would discover the tinted lights, the aroma-therapy machines, and a slew of books that claim to deliver therapy through reading and workshops. Legitimate doctors, legitimate therapists and healers, must interact with their clients. What is missing in nearly all of the theories of New Age music healing that I reviewed is personal contact. How can New Age music healers perform their services without personal contact? The rudest, most impersonal doctor must still make an occasional appearance at his client's bed.

Peter Guy Manners has managed to create a sound-healing technique in which the healer is not present, and neither is the sound. He reports,

> A woman of 60 came with a problem of generalised headaches and insomnia since being exposed in her home to low frequency noise from a large industrial cold store completed in 1977 about a quarter of a mile from her home. . . . A homeopathic pharmacist made up for her a homoeopathic potency of the low frequency noise by exposing a 50% ethanol-water mixture to the vibrations in each area for forty-eight hours. It was then made up into the 6th centesimal potency and given to the patient three times daily in tablet form. . . .
>
> The results were rapid and startling. The patient telephoned me after a fortnight to say how much better she felt. . . . After a further two weeks, practically all the symptoms had completely gone and she was forgetting to take her potency—and to think about the hum which had troubled her for so long. . . .
>
> The reader may wonder if this is indeed a homoeopathic achievement or merely the result of placebo or suggestion. In general, placebo results quickly wear off after ten to fourteen days; also, suggestion rarely reaches the depths of symptom-disturbance which this patient had and with such consistency.[15]

Mail-Order Therapists

I have unavoidably alluded to the realm of interpersonal relations throughout this book, since the field of music therapy is as rooted in this context as it is dependent upon the music. Whether a one-to-one setting or a group setting is employed, quality of interaction is of the essence. A psychotherapeutic approach in which listening represents the essence of the process is "client-centered therapy," associated primarily with the practice of Carl Rogers. Where is the "focus on the client" in Kelly and

Kenyon, Keyes, and Manners's methods? "The discipline of music therapy," writes Helen Bonny,

> concerns itself with remedial and behavioral effects of the use of carefully controlled music. Those who benefit from this therapy are inpatients and outpatients with mental and emotional disorders due to retardation, psychosocial problems and psychiatric illnesses. The music therapist works in institutions with patients in long term treatment or in schools for children with special problems. Clients with disorders such as cerebral palsy, muscular dystrophy, sensory impairments, epilepsy, birth defects and cancer have been helped. . . . The identity of the field of music therapy is changing due, in large part, to the introduction of holistic medicine and its acknowledgement that the total person—mind, body and spirit—must be brought to the "healing table." Music is the ideal instrument for this change, since it is so intimately involved in both our inner and outer lives.[16]

Note that Bonny refers to the "healing table" as a metaphor, not a concrete designation. In what way is the New Age model of healing as represented by the music healers in any way holistic or client-centered? For many New Age music healers the only view they have of their clients is in a letter or a phone call. These letters, often in the form of testimonials, are proferred as "reports," "research," "case studies," and "case examples" to support the music healers' methods and music. Mainly they are evidence of the New Age music healers' disesteem for medical science and the healing arts.

Most everyone has, at least once, bought a *National Enquirer* or *Weekly World News,* if only out of curiosity. These bastions of ethicless journalism abound with a special breed of advertisement: the testimonial ad. The July 3, 1990, *Weekly World News* contains (amidst reports of a ghost ship, an incestuous marriage, a Siamese twin giving birth to a Siamese twin, imminent UFO invasion, and a starlet's debut in the movie *Vampire Cop*) the prototypical example of an advertisement for "CAL-

BAN 3000," a miracle weight-loss pill. About a dozen "losers" testify to their success since using CAL-BAN 3000.[17] Other typical ads list scores of successful state lottery players who proclaim the virtues of particular numerologists' winning strategies. Any person of moderate intelligence will quickly question the validity of this type of come-on. The testimonial is a symptomatic feature of many quack cures and get-rich strategies. A testimonial in and of itself does not invalidate a particular nostrum, but its presence should alert us to the probability of chicanery or fraud.

Some testimonials are in the form of letters (often "unsolicited") and are frequently appended to music healers' brochures, advertisements, or even imbedded in books. In *Healing Music* Andrew Watson and Nevill Drury extend the healing properties of music into the business of real estate through a testimonial.

> Recently a friend in London presumed she had sold her home. But at the eleventh hour the sale fell through with the purchaser withdrawing. She was deeply distressed, and it was suggested she visualise the purchaser changing his mind and returning to exchange contracts. She held this visualisation over a period of three weeks, at which point the potential purchaser returned and offered her 5,000 pounds sterling more than they had agreed on in the initial instance! In all these cases the power of the image was able to rearrange circumstances. Imagine then, the results you would get from the power released when using music to accompany and transport the image.[18]

This repugnant excerpt is quite similar to the "testimonial" form of salesmanship used by various entrepreneurs in the sale of everything from miracle cures, miracle money schemes, and miracle diets to mail-order therapy.

The pages of Potentials Unlimited's brochure are crammed with testimonials. I mentioned previously their claims in regard to Jennifer Pike, the girl who suffered from "Cerebral Palsey" [*sic*] before using the company's subliminal suggestion tapes. "S. S." of Chicago writes: "I want to thank you for your *Subliminal Self-Healing* tape. I have just started playing it on a daily basis in my battle against Candida Albicans. I have not heard the whole tape while awake until the last few days. All the information that is given is so important in the healing process—coupled with your soothing voice is a great combination."[19]

I suppose that the soothing voice is not part of the "subliminal" content of the tape. To validate the testimonial as evidence, it is not unusual to find the pedigrees of testifiers included with their letter. Potentials Unlimited quotes a "T. L. T., Ph.D." of Austin, Texas: "As a clinical psychologist, I feel especially qualified to congratulate you on your fine subliminal series. The striking results that I have seen with my patients have convinced me that more education/treatment is the new trend in psychology."[20]

If T. L. T. is actually a clinical psychologist it makes no sense why he would conceal his identity. Psychologists do not conceal their treatment techniques and if he is using the subliminal tapes it would be unethical for him to do so secretively.

Patricia Joudry devotes a ten-page section of her book *Sound Therapy for the Walkman* to testimonials for the Tomatis method. (She sells Tomatis tapes, so this should not be deemed altruistic.) She allows Valerian Mayres of Saskatoon, Saskatchewan, to inform us that, "I started sound therapy because I was having a lot of trouble sleeping. Within two weeks I was sleeping very well. I also attribute to *Sound Therapy* my catch of an 8 lb. 8 oz. pickerel this summer! It is large enough to have mounted and hung in our cabin."[21]

Yes, the fish is funny, but attributing unrelated events to sound therapy is not. I do not know if Joudry would take credit for the pickerel, but taking credit for cures is endemic of most music healers. Laeh Garfield credits herself with curing Pam Lynn Pegg of cancer in two years of "healings." She reports on Pegg, a childless woman, who was "referred" to her for cervical cancer termed *carcinoma in situ* CIN III. After about an hour of other types of healing I began to Tone for her. Within a few notes I distinctly saw her as an infant, being hurled across the room head first against the wall. Immediately, I stopped and told her what I'd seen. She could barely believe it. As a baby under one year, she had no recollection of the incident. I named her father as the inflicter and the true source of her cancer. Three months later she sent me a letter saying her mother had verified that she had as an infant been dashed against a wall and wanted to know how she'd ever uncovered the information. It hadn't been her father (he'd only instigated the battering she took by being violent towards his wife, who had flung their daughter against the wall during the argument).[22]

Garfield reports that Pam Lynn "has been receiving healthy Pap tests and is now considered cancer free. Today she is alive, healthy, and still has her ability to bear children if she wishes."[23]

Garfield cured internal bleeding in a hospitalized patient: "I went to the woman's room after hours. The ward was totally chaotic, because the doctors were in the building and the nurses couldn't have me there without getting fired. Therefore, I had to work quickly. At first I did some sucking doctoring to rid the body of the poison and then Toned for about five minutes. Two days later the now healthy woman was released from the hospital."[24]

She healed a severe closed head injury: "A small child had fallen out of her grandmother's automobile . . . and it [a truck] ran over the girl's head. . . . That very day I was giving a class about healing with sound. During the section on Toning I had the class Tone for the child. I also healed her many more times using Toning, as did other people in the community. Within three weeks her head was normal."[25]

And Garfield is not hesitant to report others' stories as fact: "A student asked if I knew of any cases where Toning did the seemingly impossible. Yes, I knew of a case where a long-time quadriplegic had the use of one arm and her hand partially restored by Toning and crystal healing."[26]

Whereas legitimate books on therapy and medicine report upon treatment as a step-by-step process toward health, New Age music healing books depict evidence of quick-fix cures through music and sound such as Garfield's cures of cancer, head injury, and quadriplegia.

Physician, Hail Thyself

Sound Health by Steven Halpern and Louis Savary overflows with testimonials. Even the footnotes can be testimonials: "I was surprised and delighted to discover that Funk listed my *Zodiac Suite* among compositions having fourfold vision. I have always known that there is much more to this music than simply a relaxation response. I believe that Dr. Funk has tapped into a higher order of criticism that provides us with a glimpse into the hidden aspects of this, and much other, music."[27] This footnote testimonial is Halpern's response (I assume it is Halpern and not Savary because of the use of the personal pronoun) to a quote from the article "Music and Fourfold Vision" (revised 1983) by Joel Funk, in which Funk criticizes New Age music, which, according to Savary and Halpern, Funk feels is "not really transcendent and transpersonal."[28]

Savary and Halpern quote letters on page 165 in a chapter subsection titled "Testimony to Sound." But this is a minor quibble compared to pages of self-serving commentary on the perfection of Steven Halpern's own music. Pages 29 to 30, 43, 46 to 68, 106, 143 to 145, 179, and 184 to 186 are all lengthy encomiums to Halpern's *Spectrum Suite,* a tape that Halpern assures us is a hundred times more relaxing than the most relaxing classical music, according to his scientific testing. His perseverative salesmanship for *Spectrum Suite* is of the most frantic sort imaginable.

Halpern's *Tuning the Human Instrument* is sui generis. Of 175 pages, 10 pages (129 to 138) are testimonials. That is 6 percent of the book. Another 12 pages (139 to 150) are Halpern's self-selected reviews. That makes 13 percent of Halpern's book that is reviews of his own work, selected by himself. Such self-aggrandizing monomania is, perhaps, unprecedented. Chapter 4 (9 pages) is biographical notes cutting Halpern's tome down yet another 5 percent. Tabulating the pages, one realizes that fully 18 percent of *Tuning the Human Instrument* is about Steven Halpern. Another 33 pages (20 percent of the book) are either blank or contain no written material (such as decorative illustrations). Two pages contain nothing but addresses and a Halpern-selected discography (of only his own recordings.) Ten pages are a compilation of books Halpern recommends and eight pages are a compendium of unconnected quotes about music that Halpern has randomly assembled. Three pages make up a glossary.

So, of 175 pages, Halpern has 88 left in which to "tune the human instrument." Can he do it? Halpern's testimonials affirm that anything is possible for him, including raising the dead to exalt Halpern's name. Among his testimonials are ones from Russ Meek, director of the "Rosecrucians" [*sic*]; Eileen Deboo, a housewife; Fern Bartner, a New York choreographer; and David Allesi, a postural integrationist. Ann Haas, a "New Age distributor," writes, "My Persian cat licked itself and purred . . . after I put on your music. My fish were jumping, too."[29] (More fish testimony.) But no personal testimonial approaches the amazing example that follows the jumping fish of Ann Haas. Responding to Halpern's *Spectrum Suite,* the correspondent writes, "Truly an artistic achievement. It is like the highest form of alchemy, whereby the ephemeral has been captured for all time and rendered as an eternal expression."[30] Effusive praise, true, but the amazing part is not in the correspondent's description, but rather in the correspondent's identity; for Halpern informs us that his flattering and obsequious admirer is none other than Avicenna, the Persian philosopher and physician who sought to reconcile Aristotelian thought with Islam. Halpern reports Avicenna's occupation simply as a poet and mystic; a humble but true description nonetheless. I would be interested in seeing physical proof of Avicenna's praise of Halpern but know that there can be none. I must deny flatly Halpern's claim that Avicenna had the opportunity to hear Halpern's music and praise it, since

Avicenna died in 1037 C.E. So is Halpern pulling our leg, or is someone pulling his?

> A neighbor called on Nasrudin.
> "Mulla, I want to borrow your donkey."
> "I am sorry," said the Mulla, "but I have already lent it out."
> As soon as he had spoken, the donkey brayed. The sound came from Nasrudin's stable.
> "But Mulla, I can hear the donkey, in there!"
> As he shut the door in the man's face, Nasrudin said, with dignity: "A man who believes the word of a donkey in preference to my word does not deserve to be lent anything.[31]

The greatest threat to truth is the inability to question. Those who would lie to us have many rationales that they employ to hinder the discovery of truth. Foremost amongst the stratagems of the liars today is the attempt to deny the truth-seeker the opportunity to question. The motivations of the truth-seeker are questioned and attention is diverted from the lies. If the liar cannot succeed in diverting attention by questioning the motives of the truth-seeker, his next step is to deny the importance of reasoning about truth. He will say that it is more important to cure our ills than chop logic. This is the argument of the dishonest merchant who uses a fixed scale to weigh our purchases. As Epictetus taught, "Before the measuring of the corn we set the examination of the measure. For unless we shall first establish what is a modius [a measure of about two gallons] and what is a balance, how shall we be able to measure or weigh anything?" To the man who questions why the modius is important, Epictetus replies that the modius is important because it measures corn and logic is like the modius because "logic is that which distinguishes and investigates other things, and, as one may say, measures and weighs them."[32]

So must the seeker of the truth weigh and measure the truthfulness of those who would have power over us. Healers have power over us, sometimes power over our very lives. If one healer tells us that our disease will be cured by the application of a tone and another healer tells us that our disease can be cured only by the cutting open of our flesh, we must make a difficult decision. We must decide who we believe. Who tells us the truth? When the merchant's scale is wrong, then we must distrust him. When the New Age music healer's scale is wrong we must distrust him.

Notes

Chapter 1

1. Idries Shah, *The Pleasantries of the Incredible Mulla Nasrudin* (New York: E. P. Dutton, 1968), p. 128.

2. Peter Guy Manners, "The Principles and Practice of Cymatic Therapy, Part I," photocopy (Bretforton Hall Clinic, Worcestershire, England, n.d.), pp. 5–6.

3. Jonathan Parker's Gateways Institute, *Discoveries through Inner Quests* (Ojai, Calif.: Gateways Institute, Fall 1988), p. 22.

4. Ibid., p. 24.

5. Ruth Marks, "Sounds of Music," *The Newhall Signal*, October 24, 1986.

6. Potentials Unlimited, Inc., *Awaken* (Grand Rapids, Mich.: Potentials Unlimited, 1987), p. 2.

7. Ibid., p. 17.

8. Ibid., pp. 16–17.

9. Lawrence Huntington, *The Vulture* (Paramount, 1966), film.

10. Jonathan Goldman, "Toward a New Consciousness of the Sonic Healing Arts: The Therapeutic Use of Sound and Music for Personal and Planetary Health and Transformation," *Music Therapy: The Journal of the American Association for Music Therapy* 7, no. 1 (1988): 33.

11. Lyall Watson, *Lifetide* (New York: Simon and Schuster, 1979), pp. 147–48.

12. Ron Amundson, "The Hundredth Monkey Debunked," in *The Fringes of Reason*, ed. Ted Schultz (New York: Harmony Books, 1989), p. 181.

Chapter 2

1. Edwin A. Burtt, *The Teachings of the Compassionate Buddha* (New York: Mentor Books, 1955), p. 112.
2. Helena Petrovna Blavatsky, *Isis Unveiled* (Pasadena, Calif.: Theosophical University Press, 1972); *The Secret Doctrine* (Pasadena, Calif.: Theosophical University Press, 1974).
3. Burtt, *Teachings*, p. 63.
4. Ibid., p. 97.
5. Ibid., p. 107.
6. Helena Petrovna Blavatsky, *The Key to Theosophy* (Pasadena, Calif.: Theosophical University Press, 1946, originally published 1889), p. 13.
7. Ibid., p. 14.
8. Rudolf Steiner, *The Inner Nature of Music and the Experience of Tone* (selected lectures) (Spring Valley, N.Y.: The Anthroposophic Press, 1983), pp. 22–23.
9. Timothy Gilmore, Paul Madaule, and Billie Thompson, eds., *About the Tomatis Method* (Ontario, Canada: The Listening Centre Press, 1989).
10. Boris De Schloezer, *Scriabin: Artist and Mystic,* trans. Nicolas Slonimsky (Berkeley: University of California Press, 1987), p. 69.
11. Ibid., pp. 122–123.
12. Ibid., p. 134.
13. Aeoliah, "Harmony and the Healing Power of Music," *Halo* (Spring 1989): 14.
14. Cyril Scott, *Music* (London: Rider and Company, 1955), p. 122.
15. David Tame, *The Secret Power of Music* (Rochester, Vt.: Destiny, 1984), p. 274.
16. Scott, *Music*, p. 20.
17. Ibid., p. 21.
18. Ibid., p. 22.
19. Ibid., p. 23.

20. Ibid., p. 22.

21. Lisa Summer, "Comparing Genres of Music for Therapy," in *Music and Health Conference Proceedings* (Richmond, Ky.: Eastern Kentucky University Press, 1988), p. 97, quoting Aristotle, *On the Heavens,* trans. W. K. C. Guthrie (Cambridge, Mass.: Harvard University Press, 1960).

22. Steiner, *Inner Nature of Music,* p. 70.

23. Scott, *Music,* p. 21.

24. Steven Halpern, "Music, Harmonics, and the Tuning of the Human Instrument," paper presented at the Second National Music and Health Conference, Richmond, Ky., April 1988.

25. Jonathan Parker's Gateways Institute, *Discoveries through Inner Quests* (Ojai, Calif.: Gateways Institute, Fall 1988), p. 3.

26. Ibid., pp. 22–31.

27. Potentials Unlimited, Inc., *Awaken* (Grand Rapids, Mich.: Potentials Unlimited, 1987), p. 2.

28. Tim and Janai Lowenstein, *Gentle Places and Quiet Spaces* (Drain, Oreg.: Conscious Living Foundation, Summer 1990), p. 15.

29. Howard Richmond, "Music for Stress Reduction: Responding to the Entrainment Process," in *Music and Health Conference Proceedings* (Richmond, Ky.: Eastern Kentucky University Press, 1988), p. 145.

30. Ruth Marks, "Sounds of Music," *The Newhall Signal,* October 24, 1986, p. 8.

31. Dick Sutphen, *Master of Life* (Malibu, Calif.: Sun, 1988), 38: 17.

32. In Henry Gordon, *Channeling into the New Age* (Buffalo, N.Y.: Prometheus Books, 1988), p. 141, quoting Shirley McLaine, *Dancing in the Light* (New York: Bantam, 1985), pp. 121–22.

33. Sutphen, *Master of Life,* 38: 17.

34. "Obedience." *Obedience/On Duty,* audiocassette, (Nashville, Tenn.: Noah's Ark Productions, 1987), side A.

35. Claudia De Lys, *A Treasury of American Superstition* (New York: Bonanza, 1948), p. 438.

36. Laeh Maggie Garfield, *Sound Medicine* (Berkeley, Calif.: Celestial Arts, 1987), p. 123.

37. Ibid.

38. Ibid., p. 122.

39. Scott, *Music*, p. 73.

40. Ibid., pp. 81–82.

41. Corinne Heline, *Color and Music in the New Age* (Marina del Rey, Calif.: DeVorss, 1964), p. 79.

42. Ibid., p. 100.

43. Steven Halpern, *Tuning the Human Instrument: An Owner's Manual* (Palo Alto, Calif.: Spectrum Research Institute, 1978), pp. 32–33.

Chapter 3

1. T. W. Rolleston, trans. *Discourses of Epictetus* (New York: Home Book Company, n.d.), p. 39.

2. Rosemary Brown, *Unfinished Symphonies* (New York: Bantam Books, 1971), p. 28.

3. W. H. C. Tenhaeff, "The Phenomenon of Rosemary Brown," in liner notes to Rosemary Brown, *A Musical Seance,* Rosemary Brown and Peter Katin, Philips PHS 900–256, p. 2.

4. Ibid., p. 3.

5. "Introduction to Rosemary's Record," in liner notes to Brown, *A Musical Seance,* p. 4.

6. Aeoliah, "Harmony and the Healing Power of Music," *Halo* (Spring 1989): 11.

7. Ibid., p. 7.

8. Ibid., p. 6.

9. Ibid., p. 11.

10. Ibid., p. 12.

11. Ibid., p. 11.

12. Ibid., p. 7.

13. Ibid., p. 12.

14. Peter Guy Manners, "Cymatics" (Bretforton Hall Clinic, Worcestershire, England, n.d.), pp. 2–3.

15. Ralph Roufus, "What is Psychic Music?" brochure (Spring Valley, Calif.: Burchette Brothers), p. 1.

16. Steven Halpern, "Music, Harmonics, and the Tuning of the Human Instrument," paper presented at the Second National Music and Health Conference, Richmond, Ky., April 1988.

17. Ibid.

18. Steven Halpern, *Tuning the Human Instrument: An Owner's Manual* (Palo Alto, Calif.: Spectrum Research Institute, 1978), p. 32.

19. Laeh Maggie Garfield, *Sound Medicine* (Berkeley, Calif.: Celestial Arts, 1987), p. 41.

20. Martin Nass, "On Hearing and Inspiration in the Composition of Music," *Psychoanalytic Quarterly* 44 (1975): 434.

21. Ibid., p. 438.

22. Ibid., p. 436.

23. Ibid., p. 446.

24. Ibid., quoting Phyllis Greenacre, *The Quest for the Father. A Study of the Darwin-Butler Controversy, as a Contribution to the Understanding of the Creative Individual* (New York: International Universities Press, 1963), p. 22.

25. Ken Wilber, "The Developmental Spectrum and Psychopathology: Part II, Treatment Modalities," *Journal of Transpersonal Psychology* 16, no. 2 (1984): 146 and 147.

26. John Diamond, *The Life Energy in Music,* Vol. 2 (Valley Cottage, N.Y.: Archaeus Press, 1983), pp. 163–64.

27. Ibid. vol. 1, pp. 126–27.

28. David Tame, *The Secret Power of Music* (Rochester, Vt.: Destiny Books, 1984), p. 83.

29. Ibid., p. 84.

30. Ibid., p. 87.

31. Ibid., p. 77.

32. Charles Osborne, *Richard Wagner: Stories and Essays* (London: Peter Owen, 1973), p. 26.

33. Cyril Scott, *Music* (London: Rider and Company, 1955), p. 63.

34. Osborne, *Wagner,* p. 27.

35. Scott, *Music*, p. 63.

36. Ibid., p. 60.

37. Osborne, *Richard Wagner*, p. 134.

38. Ibid., p. 179.

39. Tame, *Secret Power*, p. 77.

40. Ibid., pp. 76–77.

41. Ibid., p. 81.

42. Scott, *Music*, p. 86.

43. Ibid., p. 86.

44. Tame, *Secret Power*, pp. 80–81.

45. Ibid., p. 98.

46. Ibid., p. 88.

47. Scott, *Music*, p. 93.

48. Garfield, *Sound Medicine*, pp. 41–42.

Chapter 4

1. Anne Feldhaus, trans., *The Deeds of God in Rodhipur* (New York: Oxford University Press, 1984), p. 95.

2. Steven Halpern, *Tuning the Human Instrument: An Owner's Manual* (Palo Alto, Calif.: Spectrum Research Institute, 1978), p. 167.

3. Steven Halpern, "Music, Harmonics, and the Tuning of the Human Instrument," paper presented at the Second National Music and Health Conference, Richmond, Ky., April 1988.

4. Donald Campbell, *The Roar of Silence* (Wheaton, Ill.: Theosophical Publishing House, 1989), pp. 109–10.

5. Rudolf Steiner, *Art as Seen in the Light of Mystery Wisdom*, trans. Pauline Wehrle and Johanna Collis (London: Rudolf Steiner Press, 1984), p. 44.

6. David Tame, *The Secret Power of Music* (Rochester, Vt: Destiny Books, 1984).

7. John Beaulieu, *Music and Sound in the Healing Arts* (Barrytown, N.Y.: Station Hill Press, 1987), p. 99.

8. Kay Gardner, *Sounding the Inner Landscape*, audiocassette (Durham, N.C.: Ladyslipper, 1990).

9. William David, *The Harmonics of Sound, Color and Vibration* (Marina del Rey, Calif.: DeVorss, 1980), pp. 100 and 14.

10. R. J. Stewart, *Music and the Elemental Psyche* (Rochester, Vt.: Destiny,

1987), p. 77. For the benefit of those readers unfamiliar with the circle of fifths, it is a construction that demonstrates the method by which the twelve pitches of Western music are determined and related in a three-to-two frequency relationship. The circle is: C, G, D, A, E, B, F♯, C♯, G♯, D♯, A♯, E♯, B♯. Note that E♯ is the same as F, and B♯ is the same as C, so that at B♯ the circle is completed. The relationship between any two successive pitches is three to two. Stewart's circle of fifths is: C, G, D, A, E, B, F, C. The relationship between the successive pitches B and F is not three to two, but rather eleven to eight, and hence a circle is not completed and five pitches are senselessly eliminated.

11. Ibid., ch. 6.

12. Joscelyn Godwin, *Harmonies of Heaven and Earth* (Rochester, Vt.: Inner Traditions International, 1987), p. 51.

13. Ibid.

14. Henry Gordon, *Channeling into the New Age* (Amherst, N.Y.: Prometheus Books, 1988), p. 168, quoting Shirley McLaine on "Larry King Live," September 10, 1985.

15. Randall McClellan, *The Healing Forces of Music* (Amity, N.Y.: Amity House, 1988), p. 69.

16. Ibid.

17. Ibid., p. 70.

18. Ibid., pp. 168–69.

19. Halpern, "Music, Harmonics, and the Tuning of the Human Instrument."

20. Halpern, *Tuning the Human Instrument*, pp. 168–69.

21. Laurel Keyes, *Toning* (Marina del Rey, Calif.: DeVorss, 1973), p. 112.

22. Nevill Drury, *Music for Inner Space* (San Leandro, Calif.: Prism Press, 1985), p. 76.

23. Andrew Watson and Nevill Drury, *Healing Music* (Garden City, N.Y.: Prism Press, 1987), p. 29.

24. Ibid., p. 29.

25. Ibid., pp. 117–20.

26. Barbara Anne Scarantino, *Music Power* (New York: Dodd, Mead, 1987), p. 195.

27. Ibid.

28. Ibid., p. 196.

29. Ibid., pp. 196–97.

30. Halpern, *Tuning the Human Instrument*, p. 153.

31. Corinne Heline, *Color and Music in the New Age* (Marina del Rey, Calif.: DeVorss, 1964), p. 75.

32. Ibid., p. 30.

33. Ibid., p. 39.

34. Ibid.

35. Ibid., p. 76.

36. Charles Osborne, *Richard Wagner: Stories and Essays* (London: Peter Owen, 1973), p. 24.

37. Ibid., p. 34.

38. Heline, *Color and Music*, pp. 89, 100.

39. Ibid., p. 89.

40. Ibid., p. 106.

41. Ibid., pp. 69–72.

42. Ibid., pp. 47 and 45.

43. Charles Boer, trans. "The Hymn to Dionysus," in *Homeric Hymns* (Dallas: Spring Publications, Inc., 1970), p. 9.

44. Heline, *Color and Music*, p. 45.

45. Kay Gardner, "Chart of Color, Sound and Energy Correspondence," in *Music and Health Conference Proceedings* (Richmond, Ky.: Eastern Kentucky University Press, 1988), p. 11. The passage regarding Kay Gardner's omission of the pitch E♭, an integral part of the chromatic scale, evident in her chart first published in 1984, was written by me in 1990 before Gardner corrected her correspondences in her 1990 publication, *Sounding the Inner Landscape*. Even though her latest book does contain the E♭, her recent musical enlightenment is proof that her original chart is a silly fabrication. This is no minor proofreading error on her part. Gardner revised her chart three years after she first constructed it and self-published it, and *still* neglected the E♭. She has yet to explain her repeated omission of E♭ in her 1987 chart revision, and her recollection of the pitch on the third go-round. Such a set of circumstances surrounding an ostensibly serious theory should lead the least skeptical reviewer to strongly doubt the foundation of the theorist's premises.

46. Corinne Heline, *Healing and Regeneration through Music* (Los Angeles: New Age Press, 1976), p. 11.

47. Ibid., p. 30.

48. Gordon, *Channeling*, quoting Shirley MacLaine on "Larry King Live," September 17, 1987.

49. Hans Cousto, *The Cosmic Octave,* trans. Christopher Baker and Judith Harrison (Mendocino, Calif.: LifeRhythm, 1988), p. 46.

50. Ibid., p. 52.

51. Ibid., p. 50.

52. Ibid., p. 44.

53. Ibid., p. 43.

54. Ibid., p. 44.

55. Heline, *Color and Music*, p. 47.

56. Godwin, *Harmonies*, pp. 158–59.

57. Jack Schwarz, *Human Energy Systems* (New York: E. P. Dutton, 1980), pp. 121–22, and 128.

58. Hal Lingerman, *Life Streams* (Wheaton, Ill.: Theosophical Publishing House, 1988), pp. 4–18.

59. Hal Lingerman, *The Healing Energies of Music* (Wheaton, Ill.: Theosophical Publishing House, 1983), p. 134.

60. Ibid., p. 123.

61. Ibid., p. 121.

62. Ibid., p. 123.

63. Ibid., p. 130.

64. Ibid., p. 187.

65. Tame, *Secret Power*, p. 238.

66. Ibid., p. 234.

67. Stewart, *Music and the Elemental Psyche*, pp. 21–22.

68. Ibid., p. 23.

69. Ibid.

70. Ibid.

71. Ibid., p. 24.

72. Ibid., pp. 24–25.

73. Ibid., p. 20.

74. Ibid., p. 36.

75. Ibid., pp. 33–34.

76. Ibid., p. 33.

77. Ibid., p. 47.

78. Godwin, *Harmonies*, p. 47 and 49, quoting Rudolf Steiner, *Vom Wesen des Musikalischen*, ed. Ernst Hagemann (Freiberg, Germany, n.p., 1974), pp. 117–26.

79. "The Tipper Gore Interview," *Nashville Musician* (n.p., 1988).

80. Halpern, *Tuning the Human Instrument*, p. 47.

81. Halpern, "Music, Harmonics, and the Tuning of the Human Instrument."

82. Steven Halpern and Louis Savary, *Sound Health* (San Francisco: Harper & Row, 1985), p. 69.

83. John Diamond, *BK Behavioral Kinesiology* (New York, NY: Harper & Row, 1979), p. 100.

84. Jeff Godwin, *Dancing with Demons* (Chino, Calif.: Chick Publications, 1988); *The Devil's Disciples* (Chino, Calif.: Chick Publications, 1985); Joscelyn Godwin, *Harmonies*.

85. Godwin, *The Devil's Disciples*, p. 87.

86. Keyes, *Toning*, pp. 113–14, from Lowell Hart, *Satan's Music Exposed* (Huntington Valley, Penn.: Salem Kirbran, n.d.).

87. Godwin, *Harmonies*, p. 51.

88. Ibid., p. 114.

89. Ibid., p. 49, quoting Rudolf Steiner, *Vom Wesen des Musikalischen*, p. 124.

90. Arthur Galston and Clifford Slayman, "Plant Sensitivity and Sensation," in *Science and the Paranormal*, ed. George Abell and Barry Singer (New York: Scribners, 1981).

91. Ibid., p. 41.

92. David, *The Harmonics of Sound*, p. 17.

93. Halpern and Savary, *Sound Health*, pp. 29–30.

94. Dorothy Retallack, *The Sound of Music and Plants* (Santa Monica, Calif.: DeVorss, 1973); Peter Tompkins and Christopher Bird, *The Secret Life of Plants* (New York: Harper & Row, 1973).

95. Godwin, *Harmonies*, p. 19.
96. Tame, *Secret Power*, pp. 143–44.
97. Ibid., p. 144.
98. Keyes, *Toning*, pp. 112–113.

Chapter 5

1. Randall McClellan, *The Healing Forces of Music* (Amity, N.Y.: Amity House, 1988),) p. 203, n. 7.

2. This is a vast oversimplification, as the "strength" of the harmonic is also weighted inversely to its distance from the fundamental; and clarinets, after the eighth harmonic begin to diverge greatly from standard, closed-tube harmonic strengths; but this is why the clarinet is a unique instrument, with a unique sound (as are all of the orchestral instruments), and not simply a "closed tube."

3. Donald Campbell, *The Roar of Silence* (Wheaton, Ill.: Theosophical Publishing House, 1989), pp. 107–108.

4. Curt Sachs, *The Wellsprings of Music* (New York: Da Capo Press, 1962).

5. R. J. Stewart, *Music and the Elemental Psyche* (Rochester, Vt.: Destiny, 1987), p. 76.

6. Sachs, *Wellsprings*, pp. 99–100.

7. Ibid., p. 104.

8. Peter Michael Hamel, *Through Music to the Self*, trans. Peter Lemesurier (Dorset, England: Element Books, 1986), p. 85.

9. Ibid., pp. 84 and 83.

10. Ibid., p. 83.

11. William David, *The Harmonics of Sound, Color and Vibration* (Marina del Rey, Calif.: DeVorss, 1980), p. 13.

12. Sachs, *Wellsprings*, p. 218.

13. Ibid., p. 219.

14. Hamel, *Through Music to the Self*, pp. 54–55.

15. Ibid., p. 99.

16. Ibid., pp. 100–101.

17. Ibid., pp. 108–109.

18. McClellan, *Healing Forces*, p. 14.

19. Ibid., p. 13.

20. Ibid., p. 16.

21. Ibid., p. 203, n. 7.

22. Dane Rudhyar, *The Magic of Tone and the Art of Music* (Boulder, Colo.: Shambhala Publications, 1982), p. 87.

23. Ibid., p. 179.

24. Ibid., p. 82.

25. Ibid., p. 55.

26. John Beaulieu, *Music and Sound in the Healing Arts* (Barrytown, N.Y.: Station Hill Press, 1987), pp. 95–96.

27. Ibid., p. 95.

28. Hermann Helmholtz, *On the Sensations of Tone*, 2d English ed., trans. Alexander J. Ellis (New York: Dover, 1954), p. 14.

29. Manly P. Hall, *The Therapeutic Value of Music Including the Philosphy of Music* (Los Angeles: Philosophical Research Society, 1982), p. 54.

30. Steven Halpern, *Tuning the Human Instrument: An Owner's Manual* (Palo Alto, Calif.: Spectrum Research Institute, 1978), p. 38.

31. Ibid.

32. Ibid., pp. 66–67.

33. Stewart, *Music and the Elemental Psyche*, pp. 134–36, quoting Gareth Knight, *The Rose Cross and the Goddess*, 1985.

34. Barbara Anne Scarantino, *Music Power* (New York: Dodd, Mead, 1987), p. 18.

35. Kay Gardner, "On Composing Medical Music," in *Music and Health Conference Proceedings* (Richmond, Ky.: Eastern Kentucky University Press, 1988), pp. 16–17.

36. Laeh Maggie Garfield, *Sound Medicine* (Berkeley, Calif.: Celestial Arts, 1987), p. 66.

37. Ibid.

38. Ibid.

39. Ibid., p. 67.

40. Ibid.

41. Ibid., pp. 67–69.

42. Kay Gardner, *Sounding the Inner Landscape* (Stonington, Maine: Caduceus Publications, 1990), p. 36.

43. Garfield, *Sound Medicine*, pp. 69–70.

44. Stewart, *Music and the Elemental Psyche*, p. 129.

45. Ibid., p. 152, n. 1.

46. Rudhyar, *The Magic of Tone*, pp. 90–91.

47. Ibid., p. 92.

48. Ibid.

49. Ibid.

50. Ibid., p. 93.

51. Ibid., pp. 97–98.

52. Ibid., p. 102.

53. Donald Campbell, "The Cutting Edge: Personal Transformation with Music," *Music Therapy: The Journal of the American Association for Music Therapy* 7, no. 1 (1988): 42–43.

54. Geoffrey Hodson, *Music Forms* (Wheaton, Ill.: Theosophical Publishing House, 1976), p. 20.

55. Campbell, *The Roar of Silence*, pp. 108–109.

56. Lisa Summer, "Comparing Genres of Music for Therapy," in *Music and Health Conference Proceedings* (Richmond, Ky.: Eastern Kentucky University Press, 1988), p. 103.

57. Gardner, "On Composing Medical Music," pp. 17–18.

58. Gardner, *Sounding the Inner Landscape*.

59. Kay Gardner, *A Rainbow Path,* audiocassette (Durham, N.C.: Lady-slipper, 1984).

60. Charles Russell Day, *The Music and Musical Instruments of Southern India and the Deccan* (Delhi, India: B. R. Publishing, 1974).

61. McClellan, *Healing Forces*, p. 82.

62. Sachs, *Wellsprings*, p. 10.

63. Ibid., pp. 10–11.

64. Beaulieu, *Music and Sound*, p. 43.

65. Rudhyar, *The Magic of Tone*, p. 59.

66. Ibid., p. 60.

67. Joscelyn Godwin, *Harmonies of Heaven and Earth* (Rochester, Vt.: Inner Traditions International, 1987), pp. 186–87.

68. Ibid., p. 167, quoting Rodney Collin, *The Theory of Celestial Influence* (London: Watkins, 1980), p. xxi.

69. Steven Halpern, "Music, Harmonics, and the Tuning of the Human Instrument," paper presented at the Second National Music and Health Conference, Richmond, Ky., April 1988.

70. Halpern, *Tuning the Human Instrument,* p. 99.

71. Ibid., p. 58.

72. Helmholtz, *On the Sensations of Tone,* ch. 5.

73. Peter Guy Manners, "Cymatics: The Structure and Dynamics of Waves and Vibrations," photocopy (Bretforton Hall Clinic, Worcestershire, England, n.d.), p. 4.

74. Ibid., p. 5.

75. Peter Guy Manners, "Penetrating One of Nature's Greatest Mysteries: The Creation of Matter by Sound," photocopy (Bretforton Hall Clinic, Worcestershire, England, n.d.), p. 6.

76. Ibid.

77. Ibid., p. 7.

78. Peter Guy Manners, "New World—Bretforton Trust," photocopy (Bretforton Hall Clinic, Worcestershire, England, n.d.), p. 4.

79. Ibid., p. 5

80. David Tame, *The Secret Power of Music* (Rochester, Vt.: Destiny, 1984), p. 216.

81. Steven Halpern and Louis Savary, *Sound Health* (San Francisco: Harper & Row, 1985), pp. 33–34, citing Lawrence Blair, *Rhythms of Vision* (New York: Schocken, 1976).

82. Ibid., p. 37.

83. David Tame, *Secret Power,* p. 217.

84. Ibid., p. 228.

85. Ibid., pp. 228–29.

86. Ibid., p. 223.

Notes to Chapter 6

1. Peter Guy Manners, "Electrobiodynamics," photocopy (Bretforton Hall Clinic, Worcestershire, England, n.d.), p. 3.

2. Jonathan Goldman, "Sonic Entrainment and the Brain," in *Music and Health Conference Proceedings* (Richmond, Ky.: Eastern Kentucky University Press, 1988), p. 37.

3. Ibid.

4. Ibid.

5. Ibid.

6. Ibid., p. 35.

7. Ibid., p. 38.

8. Ibid., pp. 36–37.

9. Steven Halpern, "Music, Harmonics, and the Tuning of the Human Instrument," paper presented at the Second National Music and Health Conference, Richmond, Ky., April 1988.

10. Jonathan Goldman, "Toward a New Consciousness of the Sonic Healing Arts: The Therapeutic Use of Sound and Music for Personal and Planetary Health and Transformation," *Music Therapy: The Journal of the American Association for Music Therapy* 7, no. 1 (1988): 29.

11. Hermann Helmholtz, *On the Sensations of Tone*, 2d English ed., trans. Alexander J. Ellis (New York: Dover, 1954), p. 8.

12. Steven Halpern, *Tuning the Human Instrument: An Owner's Manual* (Palo Alto, Calif.: Spectrum Research Institute, 1978), pp. 88 and 91.

13. Steven Halpern and Louis Savary, *Sound Health* (San Francisco: Harper & Row, 1985), pp. 38–39.

14. Ibid., pp. 32 and 37.

15. Goldman, "Sonic Entrainment," p. 46.

16. Donald Campbell, *The Roar of Silence* (Wheaton, Ill.: Theosophical Publishing House, 1989), p. 65.

17. William David, *The Harmonics of Sound, Color and Vibration* (Marina del Rey, Calif.: DeVorss, 1980), p. 65.

18. Kay Gardner, "On Composing Medical Music," in *Music and Health Conference Proceedings* (Richmond, Ky.: Eastern Kentucky University Press, 1988), p. 18, citing Olav Skille, "The Effect of Vibro Acoustic Treatment on Four Rheumatic Patients," paper presented at the International Symposium on Music and Medicine, 1984.

19. Kay Gardner and Sunwomyn Ensemble, *Garden of Ecstasy*, audiocassette (Durham, N.C.: Ladyslipper, 1989).

20. Kay Gardner, "Statement," *Music Therapy: The Journal of the American Association for Music Therapy* 8, no. 1 (1989): 118.

21. Halpern, *Tuning the Human Instrument*, p. 26.

22. Robert A. Monroe, *Journeys Out of the Body* (Garden City, N.Y.: Doubleday, 1971), p. 33.

23. Ibid., pp. 198–99.

24. Ibid., pp. 199–200.

25. Ibid., p. 258.

26. Ibid., p. 259.

27. Ibid., pp. 214–15.

28. *Monroe Institute* (Faber, Va.: The Monroe Institute, 1988), p. 9.

29. Monroe, *Journeys*, p. 266.

30. *The Monroe Institute*, p. 2.

31. Robert Sataloff, M.D., D.M.A., professor of otolaryngology, Thomas Jefferson University, written correspondence with author, 1991.

32. Helmholtz, *On the Sensations of Tone*, p. 158.

33. In discussing subjective tones one is dealing with a very subtle auditory phenomenon, which, for the most part, plays little if any role in our audition of music.

34. Sataloff, written correspondence with author, 1991.

35. *Human Plus: A System of Planned Self-Evolution* (Faber, Va.: Interstate Industries, Inc. at The Monroe Institute, 1988), p. 1.

36. Goldman, "Sonic Entrainment," p. 45.

37. Peter Guy Manners, "Brain Power—A Technology," photocopy (Bretforton Hall Clinic, Worcestershire, England, n.d.), p. 1.

38. Ibid.

39. Halpern, "Music, Harmonics, and the Tuning of the Human Instrument."

40. Dick Sutphen, *Master of Life* (Malibu, Calif.: Sun Publishing Co., 1988). 38: 27.

41. Ibid., p. 29.

42. Robert Anton Wilson, "Brain Machines Can Turn You On!" *Sound Choice* 13 (Winter 1990): 31.

43. Ibid., p. 32.

44. Ibid.

45. Goldman, "Sonic Entrainment," p. 33.

46. Wilson, "Brain Machines," pp. 31–35.

47. Ibid., p. 35.

48. Edwin A. Burtt, *The Teachings of the Compassionate Buddha* (New York: Mentor, 1955), pp. 65–66.

Notes to Chapter 7

1. Steven Halpern, *Tuning the Human Instrument: An Owner's Manual* (Palo Alto, Calif.: Spectrum Research Institute, 1978), pp. 17–18.

2. Ibid., p. 16.

3. Ibid., pp. 161–62.

4. Ibid., pp. 165–66.

5. Barbara Anne Scarantino, *Music Power* (New York: Dodd, Mead, 1987), pp. 31–32.

6. Steven Halpern and Louis Savary, *Sound Health* (San Francisco: Harper & Row, 1985), p. 46.

7. Halpern, *Tuning the Human Instrument*, p. 20.

8. Ibid., p. 45.

9. Corinne Heline, *Healing and Regeneration through Music* (Los Angeles: New Age Press, 1976), p. 20.

10. Ibid., p. 21, quoting Margaret Anderton.

11. Ibid., p. 21.

12. "Computers Bug Women, Study Finds, High Frequency Tone Doesn't Affect Men," *Nashville Tennesseean*, August 12, 1990, p. 14A.

13. Halpern, *Tuning the Human Instrument*, p. 86.

14. Halpern and Savary, *Sound Health*, p. 127, reporting on John Diamond, *Your Body Doesn't Lie* (n.p., n.d.).

15. John Diamond, *The Life Energy in Music,* vol. 1 (Valley Cottage, N.Y.: Archaeus Press, 1983), p. 89.

16. Ibid., p. 96.

17. Ibid.

18. Ibid., pp. 96–97.

19. Ibid., p. 97.

20. Ibid., pp. 97–98.

21. John Diamond, *BK, Behavioral Kinesiology* (New York: Harper & Row, 1979), pp. 102–103.

22. Diamond, *Life Energy*, pp. 89–91.

23. Ibid., p. 125.

24. Ibid., p. 13.

25. Ibid., pp. 11–12.

26. Halpern and Savary, *Sound Health*, p. 69.

27. Ibid., p. 22.

28. Ibid., p. 33.

29. Steven Halpern, "Music, Harmonics, and the Tuning of the Human Instrument," paper presented at the Second National Music and Health Conference, Richmond, Ky., April 1988.

30. Halpern, *Tuning the Human Instrument*, pp. 18–19.

31. Halpern, "Music, Harmonics, and the Tuning of the Human Instrument."

32. Ibid.

33. Ibid.

34. Howard Richmond, "Feeling Fat: A Piano Solo Composed and Performed by Howard Richmond" (Newhall, Calif.: Sound Feelings, 1984); Ruth Marks, "Sounds of Music," *The Newhall Signal* (October 24, 1986), p. 9.

35. Halpern, "Music, Harmonics, and the Tuning of the Human Instrument."

36. David Tame, *The Secret Power of Music* (Rochester, Vt.: Destiny, 1984), p. 125.

37. Ibid., pp. 125–26.

38. Ibid., p. 126.

39. Ibid., p. 262.

40. Ibid., p. 43.

41. John Diamond, *Life Energy*, vol. 2, p. 133.

42. T. W. Rolleston, trans., *Discourses of Epictetus*, (New York: Home Book Company, n.d.), pp. 52–53.

43. Patricia Joudry, *Sound Therapy for the Walkman* (St. Denis, Saskatchewan, Canada: Steele and Steele, 1984), p. 20.

44. Tame, *Secret Power*, p. 277.

45. Ibid.

46. Ibid., p. 290, referring to David A. Noebel, *The Marxist Minstrels: A Handbook on Communist Subversion of Music* (Tulsa, Okla.: American Christian College Press, 1974).

47. Manly P. Hall, *The Therapeutic Value of Music Including the Philosphy of Music* (Los Angeles: Philosophical Research Society, 1982), p. 26.

48. Peter Michael Hamel, *Through Music to the Self,* trans. Peter Lemesurier (Dorset, England: Element Books, 1986), p. 35.

49. Ibid., p. 13.

50. Ibid., p. 23.

51. Hal Lingerman, *The Healing Energies of Music* (Wheaton, Ill.: Theosophical Publishing House, 1983), p. 137.

52. Kay Gardner, "On Composing Medical Music," in *Music and Health Conference Proceedings* (Richmond, Ky.: Eastern Kentucky University Press, 1988), p. 14.

53. Ibid.

54. Hazrat Inayat Kahn, *The Music of Life* (Santa Fe, N.M.: Omega Press, 1983), pp. 343–44.

55. Ibid., pp. 341–42.

56. Cyril Scott, *Music* (London: Rider, 1955), p. 95.

57. R. J. Stewart, *Music and the Elemental Psyche* (Rochester, Vt.: Destiny, 1987), p. 42.

58. Ibid.

Notes to Chapter 8

1. T. W. Rolleston, trans. *Discourses of Epictetus* (New York: Home Book Company, n.d.), p. 208.

2. Ibid., p. 42.

3. Tom Kenyon, "Some Reflections on the Healing Power of Sound, Language, and Music: A Report on the Betar Biological Scanning System," photocopy (Lakemont, Ga.: Interdimensional Sciences, n.d.), p. 3.

4. Ibid., p. 1.

5. Ibid., p. 3. Kenyon's remark in regard to Pribram refers to Pribram's comments about the scientific method and the need for proof.

6. Ibid.

7. Ibid.

8. Ibid.

9. Ibid., p. 4.

10. Peter J. Kelly. "Biographical Data," photocopy (Lakemont, Ga.: Interdimensional Sciences, n.d.), pp. 1–2.

11. Laurel Keyes, *Toning* (Marina del Rey, Calif.: Devorss, 1973), p. 46, citing William Tiller, "Radionics, Radiesthesia and Physics," *Varieties of Healing Experiences* (Los Altos, Calif.: Academy of Parapsychology and Medicine, 1971), p. 58.

12. Ibid., pp. 48–49.

13. Ibid., p. 51.

14. Willy Ley, *Watchers of the Skies* (New York: Viking Press, 1963), p. 121.

15. "Noise That Makes You Sick," photocopy (Bretforton Hall Clinic, Worcestershire, England, n.d.), p. 1–2.

16. Helen Bonny, "Music and Healing," *Music Therapy: The Journal of the American Association for Music Therapy* 6A, no. 1 (1986): 3–4.

17. *Weekly World News,* July 3, 1990, p. 36.

18. Andrew Watson and Nevill Drury, *Healing Music* (Garden City, N.Y.: Prism Press, 1987), p. 52–53.

19. Potentials Unlimited, *Awaken* (Grand Rapids, Mich.: Potentials Unlimited, 1987), p. 13.

20. Ibid., p. 15.

21. Patricia Joudry, *Sound Therapy for the Walkman* (St. Denis, Saskatchewan, Canada: Steele and Steele, 1984), p. 139.

22. Laeh Maggie Garfield, *Sound Medicine* (Berkeley, Calif.: Celestial Arts, 1987), pp. 61–62.

23. Ibid., p. 62.

24. Ibid., pp. 59–60.

25. Ibid., p. 60.

26. Ibid.

27. Steven Halpern and Louis Savary, *Sound Health* (San Francisco: Harper & Row, 1985), p. 179 n.

28. Ibid., p. 179, citing Joel Funk, "Music and Fourfold Vision," *ReVision,* 1983.

29. Steven Halpern, *Tuning the Human Instrument: An Owner's Manual* (Palo Alto, Calif.: Spectrum Research Institute, 1978), p. 133.

30. Ibid.

31. Idries Shah, *The Pleasantries of the Incredible Mulla Nasrudin* (New York: E. P. Dutton, 1968), p. 62.

32. Rolleston, trans., *Discourses of Epictetus*, pp. 235–36.

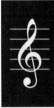

Bibliography

Abell, G. O., and B. Singer, eds. 1981. *Science and the paranormal.* New York: Scribners.

Adelman, E. 1985. Multimodal therapy and music therapy, assessing and treating the whole person. *Music Therapy: A Journal of the American Association for Music Therapy* 5 (1): 12–21.

Adorno, T. 1981. *In search of Wagner.* R. Livingstone, trans. New York: Schocken Books. (Original work published 1952.)

———. 1976. *Introduction to the sociology of music.* E. B. Ashton, trans. New York: Continuum. (Original work published 1962.)

———. 1967. *Prisms.* S. M. Weber, trans. Cambridge, Mass.: MIT Press. (Original work published 1967.)

Aeoliah. 1989. Harmony and the healing power of music. *Halo,* 4:14.

Amundson, R. 1989. The hundreth monkey debunked. In Ted Schultz, ed., *The Fringes of Reason.* New York: Harmony.

Asante, M. K. 1984. The African American mode of transcendence. *Journal of Transpersonal Psychology* 16 (2): 167–78.

Backus, J. 1969. *The acoustical foundations of music.* New York: W. W. Norton.

Beaulieu, J. 1987. *Music and sound in the healing arts.* New York: Station Hill Press.

Bentov, I. 1977. *Stalking the wild pendulum.* New York: Bantam Books.

Blavatsky, H. P. 1946. *The key to theosophy.* Covina, Calif.: Theosophical University Press.

Boer, C., trans. *Homeric hymns.* 1970. Dallas: Spring Publications.

Bonny, H. L. 1986. Music and healing. *Music Therapy: The Journal of the American Association for Music Therapy* 6A (1): 3–12.

Bonny, H. L., and L. M. Savary. 1990. *Music and your mind*. New York: Station Hill Press.

Brown, R. 1971. *Unfinished symphonies*. New York: Bantam Books.

Brother Charles. No date. *The synchronicity correspondence course/Brother Charles*. Brochure. Faber, Va.: Synchronicity Foundation.

Broucek, M. 1987. Beyond healing to "whole-ing": A voice for the deinstitutionalization of music therapy. *Music Therapy: A Journal of the American Association for Music Therapy* 6(2): 50–58.

Burchette Brothers. Form letter and order form. Spring Valley, Calif.: Author.

———. *Meditating with music instructions*. Pamphlet. Spring Valley, Calif.: Author.

———. *Psychic meditation*. Pamphlet. Spring Valley, Calif.: Author.

———. *Psychic music records*. Pamphlet. Spring Valley, Calif.: Author.

Burtt, E. A. 1955. *The teachings of the compassionate Buddha*. New York: Mentor Books.

Campbell, D. 1985. *Crystal meditations*. Audio cassette. Manhasset, N.Y.: Vital Body Marketing.

———. 1988. The cutting edge: Personal transformation with music. *Music Therapy: The Journal of the American Association for Music Therapy* 7 (1): 38–50.

———. 1989. *The roar of silence*. Wheaton, Ill.: Theosophical Publishing House.

Chailley, J. 1971. *The Magic Flute masonic opera*. H. Weinstock, trans. New York: Alfred A. Knopf. (Original work published 1968.)

Ciaffardini, D., ed. 1990. *Sound Choice* 13. Ojai, Calif.: Audio Evolution Network.

———. 1990. *Sound Choice*. 14. Ojai, Calif.: Audio Evolution Network.

Clynes, M. 1977. *Sentics*. Garden City, N.Y.: Anchor Press/Doubleday.

Cousto, H. 1988. *The cosmic octave*. C. Baker and J. Harrison, trans. Mendocino, Calif.: LifeRhythm. (Original work published 1987.)

Crandall, J. 1986. *Self-transformation through music*. Wheaton, Ill.: Theosophical Publishing House.

David, W. 1980. *The harmonics of sound, color and vibration*. Marina del Rey, Calif.: DeVorss.

Day, C. R. 1974. *The music and musical instruments of southern India and the Deccan.* Delhi, India: B. R. Publishing.

De Lys, C. 1948. *A treasury of American superstitions.* New York: Bonanza.

De Schloezer, B. 1987. *Scriabin: artist and mystic.* N. Slonimsky, trans. Berkeley: University of California Press.

Deva, B. C. 1980. *The music of India: A scientific study.* New Delhi, India: Munshiram Manoharlal Publishers.

Diamond, J. 1979. *BK, behavioral kinesiology.* New York: Harper and Row.

———. 1981–83. *The life energy in music.* 2 vols. Valley Cottage, N.Y.: Archaeus Press.

Drury, N. 1985. *Music for inner space.* San Leandro, Calif.: Prism Press.

Epictetus. *Discourses of Epictetus.* T. W. Rolleston, trans. New York: Home Book Company.

Feldhaus, A. 1984. *The deeds of God in Rodhipur.* New York: Oxford University Press.

Ferguson, M. 1980. *The Aquarian conspiracy.* New York: St. Martin's Press.

Flew, A., ed. 1987. *Readings in the philosophical problems of parapsychology.* Amherst, N.Y.: Prometheus Books.

Galston, A., and C. Slayman. 1981. Plant sensitivity and sensation. In *Science and the Paranormal.* George Abell and Barry Singer, eds. New York: Scribners. First published as The not-so-secret life of plants. May 1979. *American Scientist* 67: 337–44.

Gardner, K. 1987. *Chart of color, sound and energy correspondences.* Revised hand-written chart.

———. 1988. Esoteric concepts of music, color and healing: Workshop outline on composing medical music. *Proceedings of the Second National Conference of Eastern Kentucky University on Music and Health.* Eastern Kentucky University Press.

———. 1990. *Sounding the inner landscape.* Stonington, Maine: Caduceus Publications.

———. 1990. *Sounding the inner landscape.* Audiocassette. Durham, N.C.: Ladyslipper.

———. 1989. Statement. *Music Therapy: A Journal of the American Association for Music Therapy* 8 (1): 116–19.

Gardner, K., and Sunwomyn Ensemble. 1989. *Garden of ecstasy.* Audio cassette. Durham, N.C.: Ladyslipper.

Gardner, M. 1957. *Fads and fallacies in the name of science.* New York: Dover Publications.

Garfield, L. M. 1987. *Sound medicine.* Berkeley, Calif.: Celestial Arts.

Gateways Institute. 1987. *Discoveries through inner quests.* Brochure. Ojai, Calif.: J. Parker.

Gilmor, T., P. Madaule, and B. Thompson, eds. 1989. *About the Tomatis method.* Ontario, Canada: The Listening Centre Press.

Godwin, Jeff. 1988. *Dancing with demons.* Chino, Calif.: Chick Publications.

———. 1985. *The devil's disciples.* Chino, Calif.: Chick Publications.

Godwin, Joscelyn. 1987. *Harmonies of heaven and earth.* Rochester, Vermont: Inner Traditions International.

Goldman, J. S. 1988. Sonic entrainment and the brain. *Proceedings of the Second National Conference of Eastern Kentucky University on Music and Health.* Eastern Kentucky University Press.

———. 1988. Toward a new consciousness of the sonic healing arts: The therapeutic use of sound and music for personal and planetary health and transformation. *Music Therapy: The Journal of the American Association for Music Therapy* 7 (1): 28–33.

Gordon, H. 1988. *Channeling into the new age.* Amherst, N.Y.: Prometheus Books.

Gutman, R. 1968. *Richard Wagner: The man, his mind, and his music.* New York: Harcourt Brace Javanovich.

Haines, J. 1989. The effects of music therapy on the self-esteem of emotionally-disturbed adolescents. *Music Therapy: The Journal of the American Association for Music Therapy* 8 (1): 61–77.

Haldane, J. S. 1935. *The philosophy of a biologist,* 2d ed. Oxford: Clarendon Press.

Hall, M. P. 1982. *The therapeutic value of music including the philosphy of music.* Los Angeles: Philosophical Research Society.

Halpern, S. 1988. *Music, harmonics, and the tuning of the human instrument.* Presentation at the Second National Music and Health Conference, Richmond, Ky.

———. 1978. *Tuning the human instrument: An owner's manual.* Palo Alto, Calif.: Spectrum Research Institute.

Halpern, S., and L. Savary. 1985. *Sound health: The music and sounds that make us whole*. San Francisco: Harper & Row.

Hamel, P. M. 1986. *Through music to the self*. P. Lemesurier, trans. Dorset, England: Element Books.

Heline, C. 1964. *Color and music in the new age*. Marina del Rey, Calif.: DeVorss.

———. 1976. *Healing and regeneration through music*. Los Angeles: New Age Press.

Helmholtz, H. 1954. *On the sensations of tone*. A. Ellis, trans. New York: Dover Publications. (Original work published 1885.)

Hodson, G. 1976. *Music forms*. Wheaton, Ill.: Theosophical Publishing House.

Holroyde, P. 1972. *The music of India*. New York: Praeger Publishers.

Hutchison, M. 1989. *Human Plus: A system of planned self-evolution*. Brochure. Nellysford, Va.: Interstate Industries.

Huntington, Lawrence. *The Vulture*. Film. Paramont Pictures, 1966.

Institute for Music, Health and Education. 1990. Brochure. Boulder, Colo.: Author.

Interstate Industries, Inc. 1988. *Human plus: A system of planned self-evolution*. Brochure. Nellysford, Va.: Author.

———. 1988. *The interstate connection: The Monroe tapes*. Nellysford, Va.: Author.

Joudry, P. 1984. *Sound therapy for the walkman*. St. Denis, Saskatchewan, Canada: Steele and Steele.

Jung, C. G. 1977. *Psychology and the occult*. R. F. C. Hull, trans. Princeton, N.J.: Princeton University Press.

Karagulla, S., and D. Kunz. 1989. *The chakras and the human energy fields*. Wheaton, Ill.: Theosophical Publishing House.

Katagiri, D. 1988. *Returning to silence*. Boston: Shambhala Publications.

Keyes, L. 1973. *Toning*. Marina del Rey, Calif.: Devorss.

Khan, H. 1983. *The music of life*. Santa Fe, N.M.: Omega Press.

Ley, W. 1963. *Watchers of the skies*. New York: Viking Press.

Lingerman, H. 1983. *The healing energies of music*. Wheaton, Ill.: Theosophical Publishing House.

———. 1988. *Life streams*. Wheaton, Ill.: Theosophical Publishing House.

Lowenstein, T., and J. Lowenstein. 1978. *Gentle places and quiet spaces*. Brochure. Drain, Oreg.: Conscious Living Foundation.

Lukoff, D. 1985. The diagnosis of mystical experiences with psychotic features. *Journal of Transpersonal Psychology* 17 (2): 155–82.

Malm, W. 1977. *Music cultures of the Pacific, the Near East, and Asia.* 2d ed. Englewood Cliffs, N.J.: Prentice-Hall.

Manners, P. No date. Cymatics and its integrating phenomenon. Bretforton Scientific and Naturopathic Research Trust. Worcestershire, England: Author.

———. No date. Cymatics: The structure and dynamics of waves and vibrations. Bretforton Scientific and Medical Research Trust. Worcestershire, England: Author.

———. No date. Electrobiodynamics. Bretforton Hall Clinic. Worcestershire, England: Author.

———. No date. New world—Bretforton Trust. Bretforton Hall Clinic. Worcestershire, England: Author.

———. No date. Noise that makes you sick. Bretforton Hall Clinic. Worcestershire, England: Author.

———. No date. Penetrating one of nature's greatest mysteries: The creation of matter by sound. Bretforton Hall Clinic. Worcestershire, England: Author.

———. No date. The principles and practice of cymatic therapy. Bretforton Hall Clinic. Worcestershire, England: Author.

———. No date. Sound—Life's integrating phenomenon. Bretforton Hall Clinic. Worcestershire, England: Author.

Marks, R. October 24, 1986. Sounds of music. *The Newhall Signal.*

McClellan, R. 1988. *The healing forces of music.* Amity, New York: Amity House.

McClellan, S. 1982. *Music of the five elements.* Audiocassette. Lexington, Mass.: Spirit Records.

Monroe R. 1971. *Journeys out of the body.* Garden City, N.Y.: Doubleday.

Monroe Institute. 1989. *Are thoughts really "things"?* Pamphlet. Faber, Va.: Author.

———. 1988. *Human plus: A system of planned self-evolution.* Brochure. Faber, Va.: Interstate Industries.

———. 1988. *The Monroe Institute.* Brochure. Faber, Va.: Author.

Nash, J. R. 1976. *Hustlers and con men.* New York: M. Evans.

Nass, M. 1975. On hearing and inspiration in the composition of music. *Psychoanalytic Quarterly* 44: 431–49.

Neuman, D. 1980. *The life of music in North India.* Detroit: Wayne State University Press.

Noah's Ark Productions. 1987. *Obedience/On duty.* Audiocassette subliminal training recordings. Nashville, Tenn.: Author.

Osborne, C. 1973. *Richard Wagner: Stories and essays.* London: Peter Owen.

Potentials Unlimited, Inc. Brochure. Grand Rapids, Mich.: Author.

Priestley, M. 1988. Statement. *Music Therapy: A Journal of the American Association for Music Therapy* 7 (1): 64–67.

Retallack, D. 1973. *The sound of music and plants.* Santa Monica, Calif.: Devorss.

Richmond, H. Feeling fat: A piano solo composed and performed by Howard Richmond. Newhall, Calif.: Sound Feelings.

———. 1988. Music for stress reduction: Responding to the entrainment process. *Proceedings of the Second National Conference of Eastern Kentucky University on Music and Health.* Eastern Kentucky University.

Rollerston, T. W., trans. No date. *Discourses of Epicetus.* New York: Home Boch Company.

Roufus R. No date. *What is psychic music?* Spring Valley, Calif.: Burchette Brothers.

Rubinstein, M. 1985. *Music to my ear.* New York: Quartet Books.

Rudhyar, D. 1982. *The magic of tone and the art of music.* Boulder, Colo.: Shambhala Publications, Inc.

Sachs, C. 1962. *The wellsprings of music.* New York: Plenum Publishing.

Scarantino, B. 1987. *Music power.* New York: Dodd, Mead.

Scott, C. 1955. *Music.* London: Rider.

Schultz, T., ed. 1989. *The fringes of reason.* New York: Harmony Books.

Schwarz, J. 1980. *Human energy systems.* New York: E. P. Dutton.

Shah, I. 1968. *The pleasantries of the incredible mulla Nasrudin.* New York: E. P. Dutton.

———. 1969. *Wisdom of idiots.* New York: E. P. Dutton.

Sheldrake, R. 1981. *A new science of life.* Los Angeles: J. P. Tarcher.

Smith, F. F. 1986. *Inner bridges.* Atlanta: Humanics New Age.

Steiner, G. 1971. *In Bluebeard's castle.* New Haven: Yale University Press.

Steiner, R. 1984. *Art as seen in the light of mystery wisdom.* P. Wehrle and J. Collis, trans. London: Rudolf Steiner Press. (Original work published 1961.)

Steiner, R. 1983. *The inner nature of music and the experience of tone.* Spring Valley, N.Y.: The Anthroposophic Press.

Stewart, R. J. 1987. *Music and the elemental psyche.* Rochester, Vt.: Destiny.

Subba Rao, T. V. 1962. *Studies in Indian music.* New York: Asia Publishing House.

Summer, L. 1988. Comparing genres of music for therapy. *Proceedings of the Second National Conference of Eastern Kentucky University on Music and Health.* Eastern Kentucky University Press.

———. 1988. *Guided imagery and music in the institutional setting.* St. Louis, Mo.: MMB Music, Inc.

———. 1981. Guided imagery and music with the elderly. *Music Therapy: The Journal of the American Association for Music Therapy* 1 (1): 39–43.

———. 1989. *The hero's journey: Guided imagery and music for children.* Audio-cassette. Kansas: The Bonny Foundation.

———. 1985. Imagery and music. *Journal of Mental Imagery* 9 (4): 83–90.

———. 1995. "Unsound Medicine." In *Listening, playing, creating: Essays on the power of sound.* C. B. Kenny. Albany, N.Y.: State University of New York Press.

Sutphen, D. 1988. *Master of Life* 38. Malibu, Calif.: Sun Publishing Co.

Tame, D. 1984. *The secret power of music.* Rochester, Vt.: Destiny.

Tenhaeff, W. No date. The phenomenon of Rosemary Brown. In notes from Rosemary Brown, *A musical seance.* Recording. Rosemary Brown and Peter Katin. Philips PHS 900–256.

Tompkins, P., and C. Bird. 1973. *The secret life of plants.* New York: Harper & Row.

Watson, A., and N. Drury. 1987. *Healing music.* Garden City, N.Y.: Prism Press.

Watson, L. 1979. *Lifetide.* New York: Simon and Schuster.

Wilber, K. 1984. The developmental spectrum and psychopathology: Part II, treatment modalities. *Journal of Transpersonal Psychology* 16 (2): 137–66.

Wilson, A. Winter 1990. Brain machines can turn you on. *Sound Choice* 13: 31–35.

Winston, S. 1972. *Music as the bridge.* (Based on Edgar Cayce Readings). Virginia Beach, Va.: A.R.E. Press.

White, E. E. 1971. *Appreciating India's music.* Boston: Crescendo Publishing.

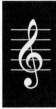

Index